After Stroke: Enhancing Quality of Life

After Stroke: Enhancing Quality of Life has been co-published simultaneously as *Loss, Grief & Care*, Volume 8, Numbers 1/2 1998.

After Stroke:
Enhancing Quality
of Life

Wallace Sife, PhD
Editor

After Stroke: Enhancing Quality of Life has been co-published simultaneously as *Loss, Grief & Care*, Volume 8, Numbers 1/2 1998.

The Haworth Press, Inc.
New York • London

After Stroke: Enhancing Quality of Life has been co-published simultaneously as *Loss, Grief & Care,* Volume 8, Numbers 1/2 1998.

The development, preparation, and publication of this work has been undertaken with great care. However, the publisher, employees, editors, and agents of The Haworth Press and all imprints of The Haworth Press, Inc., including The Haworth Medical Press and Pharmaceutical Products Press, are not responsible for any errors contained herein or for consequences that may ensue from use of materials or information contained in this work. Opinions expressed by the author(s) are not necessarily those of The Haworth Press, Inc.

The Haworth Press, Inc., 10 Alice Street, Binghamton, NY 13904-1580 USA

Cover design by Thomas J. Mayshock Jr.

Library of Congress Cataloging-in-Publication Data

After stroke : enhancing quality of life / Wallace Sife.
    p. cm.
    "After stroke : enhancing quality of life has been co-published simultaneously as Loss, grief & care, Volume 8, numbers 1/2, 1998."
    Includes bibliographical references and index.
    ISBN 0-7890-0321-X (alk. paper).–ISBN 0-7890-0341-4 (alk. paper)
    1. Cerebrovascular disease–Patients–Rehabilitation. 2. Cerebrovascular disease–Patients. I. Sife, Wallace. II. Loss, grief & care. vol. 8, no. 1-2, 1998.
RC388.5.A36 1998   98-16152
616.8′1–dc21   CIP

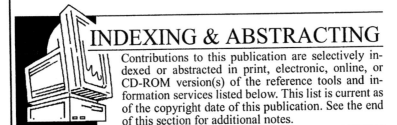

INDEXING & ABSTRACTING

Contributions to this publication are selectively indexed or abstracted in print, electronic, online, or CD-ROM version(s) of the reference tools and information services listed below. This list is current as of the copyright date of this publication. See the end of this section for additional notes.

- *Abstracts of Research in Pastoral Care & Counseling,* Loyola College, 7135 Minstrel Way, Suite 101, Columbia, MD 21045

- *Academic Abstracts/CD-ROM,* EBSCO Publishing Editorial Department, P.O. Box 590, Ipswich, MA 01938-0590

- *AgeInfo CD-Rom,* Centre for Policy on Ageing, 25-31 Ironmonger Row, London EC1V 3QP, England

- *Applied Social Sciences Index & Abstracts (ASSIA) (Online: ASSI via Data-Star) (CDRom: ASSIA Plus),* Bowker-Saur Limited, Maypole House, Maypole Road, East Grinstead, West Sussex RH19 1HH, England

- *CINAHL (Cumulative Index to Nursing & Allied Health Literature), in print, also on CD-ROM from CD PLUS, EBSCO, and SilverPlatter, and online from CDP Online (formerly BRS), Data-Star, and PaperChase. (Support materials include Subject Heading List, Database Search Guide, and instructional video),* CINAHL Information Systems, P.O. Box 871/1509 Wilson Terrace, Glendale, CA 91209-0871

- *CNPIEC Reference Guide: Chinese National Directory of Foreign Periodicals,* P.O. Box 88, Beijing, People's Republic of China

- *Communication Abstracts,* Temple University, Communication Sciences Dept., Weiss Hall, Philadelphia, PA 19122

- *Family Studies Database (online and CD/ROM),* National Information Services Corporation, 306 East Baltimore Pike, 2nd Floor, Media, PA 19063

- *Health Source: Indexing & Abstracting of 160 selected health related journals, updated monthly,* EBSCO Publishing, 83 Pine Street, Peabody, MA 01960

- *Health Source Plus: expanded version of "Health Source" to be released shortly,* EBSCO Publishing, 83 Pine Street, Peabody, MA 01960

(continued)

- *IBZ International Bibliography of Periodical Literature,* Zeller Verlag GmbH & Co., P.O.B. 1949, d-49009 Osnabruck, Germany

- *INTERNET ACCESS (& additional networks) Bulletin Board for Libraries ("BUBL"), coverage of information resources on INTERNET, JANET, and other networks.*
  - <URL:http://bubl.ac.uk/>
  - The new locations will be found under <URL:http://bubl.ac. uk/link/>.
  - Any existing BUBL users who have problems finding information on the new service should contact the BUBL help line by sending e-mail to <bubl@bubl.ac.uk>.
  The Andersonian Library, Curran Building, 101 St. James Road, Glasgow G4 0NS, Scotland

- *Leeds Medical Information,* University of Leeds, Leeds LS2 9JT, United Kingdom

- *Mental Health Abstracts (online through DIALOG),* IFI/Plenum Data Company, 3202 Kirkwood Highway, Wilmington, DE 19808

- *New Literature on Old Age,* Centre for Policy on Ageing, 25-31 Ironmonger Row, London EC1V 3QP, England

- *Referativnyi Zhurnal (Abstracts Journal of the All-Russian Institute of Scientific and Technical Information),* 20 Usievich Street, Moscow 125219, Russia

- *Sage Family Studies Abstracts (SFSA),* Sage Publications, Inc., 2455 Teller Road, Newbury Park, CA 91320

- *Sapient Health Network,* 720 SW Washington Street #400, Portland, OR 97205-3537

- *Social Planning/Policy & Development Abstracts (SOPODA),* Sociological Abstracts, Inc., P.O. Box 22206, San Diego, CA 92192-0206

- *Social Work Abstracts,* National Association of Social Workers, 750 First Street NW, 8th Floor, Washington, DC 20002

- *Sociological Abstracts (SA),* Sociological Abstracts, Inc., P.O. Box 22206, San Diego, CA 92192-0206

(continued)

SPECIAL BIBLIOGRAPHIC NOTES

related to special journal issues (separates)
and indexing/abstracting

- ❑ indexing/abstracting services in this list will also cover material in any "separate" that is co-published simultaneously with Haworth's special thematic journal issue or DocuSerial. Indexing/abstracting usually covers material at the article/chapter level.

- ❑ monographic co-editions are intended for either non-subscribers or libraries which intend to purchase a second copy for their circulating collections.

- ❑ monographic co-editions are reported to all jobbers/wholesalers/approval plans. The source journal is listed as the "series" to assist the prevention of duplicate purchasing in the same manner utilized for books-in-series.

- ❑ to facilitate user/access services all indexing/abstracting services are encouraged to utilize the co-indexing entry note indicated at the bottom of the first page of each article/chapter/contribution.

- ❑ to facilitate user/access services all indexing/abstracting services are encouraged to utilize the co-indexing entry note indicated at the bottom of the first page of each article/chapter/contribution.

- ❑ this is intended to assist a library user of any reference tool (whether print, electronic, online, or CD-ROM) to locate the monographic version if the library has purchased this version but not a subscription to the source journal.

- ❑ individual articles/chapters in any Haworth publication are also available through the Haworth Document Delivery Service (HDDS).

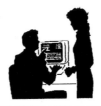

ABOUT THE EDITOR

Wallace Sife, PhD, is a published poet, humanist, and psychologist in private clinical practice in Brooklyn, New York. He has specialized in learning disorders, holistic behavior modification, poetry therapy, and biofeedback. Dr. Sife is currently at the forefront in developing the field of pet bereavement, and writes in a wide number of other areas.

After Stroke:
Enhancing Quality of Life

CONTENTS

PART II: PROFESSIONAL CONTRIBUTIONS

Introduction

Wallace Sife

Every good book has a complex personality of its own. This symposium offers a collective wisdom that is unique in the literature of stroke. Before its birth, it seemed to grow of its own direction through several major developmental stages.

In its embryonic phase, when I first began reading the many varied manuscripts, long and short, that had been submitted, I had hoped to put together a fine collection of the most enlightening recent experiences and developments in the world of stroke. But, in reading all these separate accounts together, I was struck by two persistent themes that seemed to be crying out for attention. Indeed, they all can be seen as inspirational. The incipient book had already begun to define itself in ways I could not have realized, if not seen in this new perspective. I was also impressed by the fact that every contributor expressed a personal passion. Depending on the viewpoint, in different ways they each attested to two truths: that the dedicated professional does make a difference by being both a caregiving unique person and a healer; and second, that the human spirit is free, and is not limited or defined by physical bonds or traditional thinking.

Stroke tyrannically redefines everything. When confronted by its terrible ultimatum it could cause either the downfall or the rebirth of the survivor. It forces him to either accept responsibility for his existence in the newly flawed body, or sink into despair and utter personal destruction.

Wallace Sife, MA, PhD, MS, is a published poet, humanist and a psychologist in private clinical practice in Brooklyn, NY. He has specialized in learning disorders, holistic behavior modification, poetry therapy and biofeedback. Dr. Sife is currently at the forefront in developing the field of pet bereavement, and writes in a wide number of other areas.

[Haworth co-indexing entry note]: "Introduction." Co-published simultaneously in *Loss, Grief & Care* (The Haworth Press, Inc.) Vol. 8, No. 1/2, 1998, pp. 1-6; and: *After Stroke: Enhancing Quality of Life* (ed: Wallace Sife) The Haworth Press, Inc., 1998, pp. 1-6. Single or multiple copies of this article are available for a fee from The Haworth Document Delivery Service [1-800-342-9678, 9:00 a.m. - 5:00 p.m. (EST). E-mail address: getinfo@haworth.com].

We have the choice of being victim or survivor, and must claw our own way through a horrific odyssey in an existential struggle for personal redefinition. But through it all, the human spirit soars and sings.

This concept of personal renewal and redemption is not new or unique. It is richly reflected in folklore, literature, and religion. The theme of rebirth, of rising from one's own ashes, is as old as recorded history. But, like so many other things in life, it remains underexamined as a means for self-improvement. This, however, may be the ideal metaphor for stroke survivors, and will be discussed in greater detail later.

One of the greatest roles one can undertake is as a healer. This marvelous opportunity can be approached in many possible ways–as every chapter in this book demonstrates so well. The professional healers who have contributed to this volume are experienced authorities, and range in specialty, from medical doctors, nurses, psychologists, and the whole spectrum of practitioners and therapists, specially trained to work with survivors of stroke. Each one has an important message to give, about the latest developments being made in the treatment of stroke. Their dedicated professionalism is as inspiring as their messages are informative. The treatments for stroke have made significant progress in the last few years, and these specialists have much to tell us.

Several of the contributors to this book are survivors of stroke. They each made it the hard way through this hellish experience, and now they want to help others heal themselves. There is so much that they have learned from this ordeal, and each has a passion to teach others how to be reborn out of the horrors of stroke. Theirs are living stories of terrible adversity, hope, achievement and personal fulfillment. They have come out of the shadow of the valley of death, to inspire us with their struggles and successes.

It is fascinating to find closely related themes in these personal accounts. In different ways, these stroke survivors discovered the same truths about survival. On reading these accounts together, the common denominators they found yield valuable insights, hidden deep within the stroke experience. But to discover this, it was necessary to assemble them as a synthesis. Each of these people found it important to serve as a healer to others who have suffered stroke–or their caregivers and professional practitioners.

This book is designed for anyone who has an interest in what the stroke experience means. This includes stroke survivors, caregivers, friends and family, as well as the entire family of professionals who work with these people. From the collected wisdom of our authors comes a heightened knowledge and understanding. It is a comprehensive clearing out of cobwebs, misinformation, and outdated knowledge. It offers so much, in so many ways. But like everything else, whatever benefits one gains from reading this are waiting to be discovered.

NATIONAL STROKE AND QUALITY OF LIFE MEDICAL EDUCATION INSTITUTE (NSEI)

A Division of The American Institute of Life-Threatening Illness and Loss

MISSION, GOALS, AND PROGRAM

MISSION STATEMENT

To assist stroke-affected people in their search for an acceptable quality of life–by offering vital medical advice, practical survivor techniques, and information about resources which have proven to be helpful to others.

To make every effort to instill in medical personnel preparing to enter the stroke field, the sensitivity required when dealing with those struggling to overcome long-term affliction.

To involve medical professionals in approaches to restoring stroke survivor quality of life.

To focus medical professional attention on post-stroke quality of life issues.

To focus medical education on approaches to restoring stroke survivor quality of life.

To incorporate an awareness of post-stroke quality of life issues in the medical curriculum.

OVERVIEW

The National Stroke and Quality of Life Medical Education Institute (NSEI) has been an outgrowth of the development and implementation over a period of two years of the symposium "Stroke and Quality of Life: Psychosocial Adaptation to Loss and the Bereavement of Physical Disability," which was held March 9-11, 1994, and the deliberations of the multidisciplinary group responsible for the symposium and post-symposium planning.

In inaugurating the Education Institute, The American Institute has furthered its principal mission–that of offering guidance and assistance to caregiving efforts of members of all of the multi-disciplinary fields involved in caring for life-threatened stroke patients and their families. The American Institute's goal is to maximize the quality of life of those to whom the team ministers. These interests in the stroke area span private practice, clinical teams, the medical center, the corporate world, the media, health care delivery organizations and regulatory groups, as well as organizations that serve the pharmaceutical industry, consumer and patient advocacy groups, and government.

The Education Institute was organized to help provide structure for and implement change in the field of stroke caregiving as, related to quality of life–at crucial focal points in the stroke health care delivery system.

EDUCATION INSTITUTE SPONSORSHIP

The National Stroke and Quality of Life Medical Education Institute (NSEI) is sponsored by the American Institute of Life-Threatening Illness and Loss, a division of the Foundation of Thanatology, which is based at Columbia-Presbyterian Medical Center, in the Department of Psychiatry of the College of Physicians and Surgeons, Columbia University. The Education Institute also has the sponsorship of other important units of the Columbia-Presbyterian Medical Center. In addition, selected organizations, school groups, and services outside the Columbia family are, as with other American Institute projects, being sought as ongoing, co-sponsors.

The overall activities of the American Institute have spanned more than 25 years and have been devoted to developing programs for improved and positive approaches to the care of patients and families facing a wide variety of life-threatening illnesses and losses–activities which have resulted in our series of two and three-day interdisciplinary symposia, as well as some 128 full-length texts–since 1969. The Stroke Symposium was the 108th in the series.

EMPHASIS AT THE NATIONAL LEVEL

A major priority of Education Institute activity will deal with efforts to raise the consciousness of society on stroke and quality of life issues–efforts designed to alter the course of the impact of this life-threatening and person-threatening illness on patients and families, for generations to come.

HISTORICAL ASPECTS

Those already involved with the symposium and the early origins of the Education Institute have been gratified by the favorable acceptance response of others in the field more peripherally associated with the planning phases of the symposium and initial planning activities for the Education Institute.

As their first effort, members and others interested in becoming members, and/or those interested in the Education Institute for any reason, are asked to review an initial compilation of the many excellent suggestions for conferences and activities of the Education Institute which have been suggested to date. They are also requested to rate the items in roughly the order of priority in which they might be considered for implementation. Additional suggestions would be greatly valued. This simple step, in which all are participating, is crucial to further planning.

No membership dues in the Education Institute are involved. Academic and clinical expertise and assistance are needed, not personal funding.

STROKE EDUCATION INSTITUTE PUBLICATIONS

The papers from conferences are to be published in volumes representing the publication effort of the NSEI.

A substantial number of publication directions are being explored, since this avenue is seen as a primary area of educational activity of the NSEI.

MEDICAL STUDENT EDUCATION CONFERENCE SERIES

The four-year stroke medical student education conference series is sponsored by the Education Institute, its ongoing sponsors, and by selected other academic institutions, departments and/or committees of these–as well as by such corporate groups as may be appropriate.

A state-of-the-art consensus conference will be held to meet the challenges of stroke and quality of life issues, as well as medical student education in the areas of stroke. This includes the development of multiple tracks concerned with a curriculum, a primer for medical students, teaching instruments designed for this area of medical expertise, a clearing house for teaching materials, approaches to evaluation of teaching programs, and the development of a national stroke medical school faculty cadre, from virtually every medical school in the country, to work with and to implement the programs and outcomes.

PATIENTS AND FAMILY INVOLVEMENT

Central to the effective operation of the NSEI is its Patient and Family Committee (including its outreach program to the general public). The 1994 symposium has already provided a much needed and rich forum in an academic setting for the launching of the work of the Patient and Family Committee.

FUNDING

All involved in the work of the NSEI are asked to be helpful in obtaining sources of funding in-kind materials, and services to assist the operation of the NSEI.

Address Correspondence to

National Stroke and Quality of Life Medical Education Institute
A Division of The American Institute of Life-Threatening Illness and Loss
Columbia-Presbyterian Medical Center
630 West 168th Street
New York, NY 10032
(212) 928-2066

Dr. Austin H. Kutscher, Administrative Chair

The National Stroke and Quality of Life Medical Education Institute is a Division of The American Institute of Life-Threatening Illness and Loss.

PART I
CLINICAL PERSPECTIVES

Pathophysiology of Stroke

Fletcher McDowell

The term "stroke" is an ancient one. If you look it up in the *Oxford English Dictionary* it has 20 different meanings. These include: a stroke of lightning, a stroke of the pen, a stroke of an oar, a stroke of luck. But it also came to mean any kind of cataclysmic event that occurred to a human being. In ancient times it included everything that we now recognize as stroke but also included seizures and fainting spells.

It has been only in the last hundred years that stroke has become understood and sorted out into its various entities. It's not a unified diagnosis as there are a number of different causes, each of which has a different pathology, different treatments and different frequencies, incidence and prevalence. These include cerebral infarction or ischemic stroke, intracerebral hemorrhage and subarachnoid hemorrhage. These names do not imply causation but provide a useful clinical classification.

The most common reason for stroke is cerebral infarction, which is due

Fletcher McDowell, MD, is Executive Medical Director, Burke Rehabilitation Hospital, 785 Mamarinack Avenue, White Plains, NY 10605.

[Haworth co-indexing entry note]: "Pathophysiology of Stroke." McDowell, Fletcher. Co-published simultaneously in *Loss, Grief & Care* (The Haworth Press, Inc.) Vol. 8, No. 1/2, 1998, pp. 7-13; and: *After Stroke: Enhancing Quality of Life* (ed: Wallace Sife) The Haworth Press, Inc., 1998, pp. 7-13. Single or multiple copies of this article are available for a fee from The Haworth Document Delivery Service [1-800-342-9678, 9:00 a.m. - 5:00 p.m. (EST). E-mail address: getinfo@haworth.com].

to death of brain tissue caused by decreased or absent blood supply to a part or all of the brain for a long enough period so that brain tissue dies. Cerebral hemorrhage means that a blood vessel has broken inside of the brain, and caused bleeding into the brain, usually with formation of a large clot creating a hematoma within the brain. This can destroy and compress brain tissue and cause dysfunction. Subarachnoid hemorrhage, is bleeding over the surface of the brain, usually from a rupture of an aneurysm on one of the large arteries at the base of the brain. The frequencies of these diagnoses is quite different. Cerebral infarction causes about 80% of all strokes, cerebral hemorrhage 12% and subarachnoid hemorrhage 8%. The clinical characteristics of these particular entities of stroke are quite unique.

For cerebral infarction, the brain is deprived of blood flow, either total or locally. If this continues 10 minutes or longer, there is conspicuous change in nervous system function. After 10 seconds of decreased blood supply in the entire brain individuals faint. If the decrease is local and if the blood supply is not restored quickly, the area the brain supplies dies. Most strokes are due to local impairment of blood supply on one side of the brain or another on the posterior portion of the brain. This is most commonly due to obstruction of an artery supplying the brain. Obstruction is most often due to atherosclerosis. This is an extremely common condition, and is almost universal. In fact the evidence suggests that less than 4% of the people in our population die without some evidence of extensive atherosclerotic disease. It is common, but not everybody with atherosclerosis has a stroke. In addition to atherosclerotic obstruction of arteries, clots can form in the heart or in the vessels leading to the brain. These can break off and travel downstream and plug vessels. This is probably as common a cause for stroke as mechanical obstruction of arteries by atherosclerosis.

When a stroke occurs from decreased blood supply to a particular portion of the brain, the most common result is weakness, loss of sensation, and sometimes visual impairment on the side of the body opposite to the brain infarction. The victim has paralysis or weakness of the face, hand, arm and leg as well as a sensation of numbness and sensory loss on the same side. Strokes that are due to impairment of blood supply of the posterior portion of the brain have a wide variety of clinical possibilities. They most often cause some degree of paralysis on one side or both sides of the body, with loss of sensation, changes in the ability of controlling movements, and often some impairment of eye movement. If brain infarction occurs in the dominant hemisphere, which in most people is the left cerebral hemisphere, stroke victims will have some difficulty in understanding language or speaking. Combinations of impaired speech production and understanding are most common. With a *large* stroke, which involves the right cerebral hemisphere, victims may have major problems with awareness of the world on one side of the body or another. They also may be unaware of being paralyzed or that the left side of their body exists.

The physical impairment caused by stroke tends to improve over time. Generally, the improvement that occurs is most evident in the first three months after stroke, and is most evident in the lower extremities. Skilled hand and finger movements rarely return to normal, and most persons with a stroke report that despite near normal return of function they are never really back to the level of function they had before. If a concert pianist has a stroke, regardless of how much recovery occurs, it is unlikely that performance will return to the prestroke level. Virtually anyone who has had a stroke, and can talk about their experience, will tell you that they are never the same person following the stroke. Generally, infarction occurs rather abruptly, sometimes with warning signs briefly suggesting that a stroke is going to happen. These warning signs may last for ten to twenty minutes. They are strong indications that a stroke may occur.

Patients with intracerebral hemorrhage usually have a rather abrupt change in function, with headache and weakness developing on one side of the body. If the hemorrhage is large enough to compress of the brain stem, patients will lose consciousness. The sequence of events is sometimes not always abrupt, and symptoms may gradually develop over a period of hours. Generally intracerebral hemorrhage, when it occurs, produces an acute event over a period of a few hours. It almost never has warning signs suggesting that it's going to happen. The diagnosis of intracerebral hemorrhage is easily made by the CT scan, which clearly displays bleeding into the brain. CT scanners are now available in about 90% of the hospitals, in the United States.

Determining whether a stroke is due to changes in cerebral blood flow or hemorrhage is vitally important because treatment of cerebral infarction often involves medication, which increases the chances of bleeding. The mortality of intracerebral hemorrhage is extremely high, depending on how large the hemorrhage is and whether the victim loses consciousness. Mortality from intracerebral hemorrhage can be as high as 70-80%. Small hemorrhages in the brain are not associated with high mortality but they do cause impairment of function. Some hemorrhages resolve without permanent changes in nervous system function.

Subarachnoid hemorrhage is a unique kind of stroke and easily identified if information about the onset is available. Usually, a victim of subarachnoid hemorrhage will report the abrupt onset of a severe headache, usually described as the most severe headache they have ever had. It is so intense that it stops a patient's normal daily function. Many people have headache and manage it with aspirin and go to work, but usually not the headache of subarachnoid hemorrhage. At times the onset of subarachnoid hemorrhage may be associated with a brief period of loss of consciousness. If there is bleeding from the aneurysm into the brain there may be weakness on one side of the body or another. Because blood is an irritant around the outside of the brain, after several hours patients will have a stiff neck. On CT scanning which should be done for all patients suspected of having a subarachnoid hemorrhage, there will be evidence of bleeding over the surface of the brain. If that is found, the next procedure is to perform cerebral angiography to determine the source of the bleeding. Most commonly, it is a ruptured aneurysm found on one of the large cerebral arteries at the base of the brain, including the internal carotid, the middle cerebral or the anterior cerebral artery. The mortality of subarachnoid hemorrhage is high. It varies from 30 to 40% for the initial hemorrhage. A serious problem for victims of subarachnoid hemorrhage is recurrent bleeding. And each recurrence carries the same risk of mortality. Recurrence occurs in about 35-40% of patients. Because blood is an irritant and is found over the surface of the brain in contact with cerebral arteries, it often reduces the caliber of arteries supplying the brain or vasospasm. This occurs several days after the onset and is associated with another increase in mortality. It can decrease cerebral blood flow, and often causes cerebral infarction. It is extremely important to deal with the bleeding source, to be sure that recurrent bleeding is prevented. This should be done as quickly as possible. Unfortunately, many of those who survive subarachnoid hemorrhage have enough brain destruction to suffer permanent impairment, both in intellect and motor function.

Mortality in cerebral infarction is generally about 20%, but the frequency of disability is as high as about 40%, in stroke survivors. For intracerebral hemorrhage, mortality can vary from 45-70% and the disability can be very high. Subarachnoid hemorrhage mortality is high, but disability can be moderate. Many victims of subarachnoid hemorrhage survive without evidence of neurological impairment.

An important question is how frequently stroke occurs. This is done by calculating its incidence and prevalence. Incidence is an important determination for epidemiologists, and indicates how many individuals in a given population have a stroke in a given period of time. This is expressed as the annual number of strokes occurring in a population of 100,000 per year. There is difficulty getting this kind of information because it is necessary to have a static population living in a community for one year. Accurate medical records must be kept of how many new strokes have occurred in that population. The reported incidence in the USA is about 100-150/100,000.

Stroke is an age-related condition. Its incidence rises with age from age 55 onwards, doubling every decade. The chances of having a stroke are greatly increased after an individual reaches age sixty. The incidence of stroke has been falling since 1948 from about 200 per 100,000 population down to around 100 per 100,000 in the late 1980s. There was a slight increase in incidence in the late 1980s, which is thought possibly due to the more accurate identification of victims of stroke, using CT scans. Most of the data on incidence come from studies done at the Mayo Clinic, using the population around the clinic in Olmstead County, Minnesota. The population there is fairly stable, with the medical care level quite high, and the medical record keeping excellent. These data are not necessarily applicable to other areas in the United States. There are other major factors influencing areas such as the southeastern part of the country, or those with certain minority populations, such as the district around the Columbia Presbyterian Hospital, in New York City.

For stroke there has been a steady decline in age adjusted mortality. It has come down to about one-half, from about 100 per 100,000 population in 1950 to about 50 per 100,000 in 1980. The mortality decline is most evident in the older age groups.

Another important determination is prevalence of stroke. This refers to the number of stroke survivors in a given population. Prevalence data is based on studies from the Mayo Clinic and other centers, which report an age adjusted rate of 612 per 100,000. This rate is age-related so that for individuals aged 55-64 the rate is 810. For those aged 65-74 it is 3560, and for persons over age 75 it is 5970. As the population of the United States ages and the mortality from stroke declines, there will be an increase in numbers of disabled individuals with stroke, requiring care. About 40% of all stroke victims have significant physical disability. To give an idea of the size of the problem, using a population of one million people, each year there would be about 108 cases of subarachnoid hemorrhage, and 1000 cases of stroke. Of these, 831 would be cerebral infarctions and the rest cerebral hemorrhages.

Risk factors for stroke have been extensively studied. Those such as age, sex, heredity, and diabetes are unchangeable. Others, such as hypertension, smoking, diet and daily habits, can be changed. Hypertension has been identified as the most important risk factor for intracerebral hemorrhage, and a very significant one for ischemic stroke. With treatment of high blood pressure the risk of intracerebral hemorrhage has declined significantly. Because hypertension accelerates the development of atherosclerosis, control of both systolic and diastolic hypertension has been shown to decrease the frequency and incidence of cerebral infarction.

Diabetes is a common cause of increased atherosclerotic disease. This can not be cured, but information is building that careful diabetic control reduces the chances of complications related to the development of atherosclerosis. This indicates a reduction in the chances of stroke.

Heart disease is an important risk factor for stroke especially if there is atrial fibrillation, a history of myocardial infarction or congestive heart failure. The main underlying cause of heart disease and stroke is atherosclerosis. This has a distinct timetable for development in various parts of the circulation. The process starts when there is atherosclerosis of the aorta. In one's twenties it already can be found in the coronary arteries, and by the third decade it is beginning to develop in arteries leading to the brain. When an individual reaches age 50 to 60 it often becomes symptomatic. The most common result is myocardial infarction. It is almost certain that when an individual has a stroke, he also has significant coronary artery disease, although it may not be symptomatic.

Another important risk factor is the occurrence of brief episodes of weakness or sensory loss on one side of the body, with or without some difficulty with vision or speaking. These episodes are brief, and have been called transient ischemic attacks. They last from a few minutes to a few hours and leave the individual with no residual deficits. They are examples of what might occur if a permanent stroke occurred. Although the symptoms and signs disappear, brain scans will often reveal evidence of small cerebral infarctions. The reported frequency of these attacks is variable, depending on how the problem is studied. But it is believed that about 1/3 of the patients who have stroke have had these attacks before. Their occurrence definitely indicates that there has been a brief change in the cerebral circulation, either due to an embolus blocking a small vessel or to a local reduction in cerebral blood flow because of obstruction in a cerebral vessel. The fact that they have occurred is a very strong predictor that an individual may be likely to have a stroke. Not everyone with a transient ischemic attack will have a stroke, but the frequency of stroke in those who have these attacks is high, making this is an important risk factor.

Cigarette smoking has been connected with coronary artery disease and the occurrence of stroke. Those who smoke have a higher risk of having stroke and heart attack than those who don't. The evidence is good that if individuals stop smoking the chances of having a stroke are reduced. Also alcohol and drug abuse are recognized as a cause of stroke, especially in younger individuals.

Elevated blood lipids have been shown to be associated with the development of atherosclerosis and coronary artery disease. They probably have some effect on the development of cerebral artery disease. Most of those with serious problems with elevated lipids have heart disease before they have stroke. Genetic and hereditary factors are being investigated, and are believed to have considerable influence on the chances of developing stroke.

An extremely important issue has become significant because of new developments in the treatment of stroke. This is the advisability of starting treatment as soon as possible after the onset of symptoms suggesting the possibility of stroke. It is suggested that if begun within three to six hours after onset of symptoms, stroke may be avoided, or the amount of brain damage and residual dysfunction can be reduced. This may mean that a person who starts having symptoms of stroke must be in treatment within 90 minutes to two hours. Symptoms suggesting a stroke must be viewed with the same urgency as those which suggest the onset of a heart attack. As yet, we are not accustomed to doing that for patients with threatened stroke. The attitude has been that if one has symptoms suggesting a stroke, usually a physician may advise the person to lie down and take an aspirin. And if symptoms are present the next day, it's a stroke. If one is free of these symptoms in a few minutes, it may be only a transient ischemic attack. This attitude must change if stroke is to be prevented and the disability associated with stroke is to be avoided or reduced.

The Psychiatry of Stroke

D. Peter Birkett

If stroke only caused paralysis and a danger of death it would still be a terrible affliction. Yet the biggest tragedy of stroke lies in its mental effects. And most of the disability it produces is mental, rather than physical. There has been some tendency to ignore the psychiatric aspects of stroke in the past, perhaps because chronic long-term illness affecting the elderly was not then a focus of medical attention.

DEFINITION

Psychiatric interest in stroke begins with the question of definition. The World Health Organization defines stroke as a vascular lesion of the brain, resulting in a neurologic deficit, persisting for more than 24 hours or resulting in death. There are several other official definitions and classifications. They mostly ignore mental symptoms.

The new imaging methods such as the CAT scan and magnetic resonance imaging (MRI) have led to the realization that many patients with purely mental symptoms have brain infarcts. People with brain infarcts with no non-psychiatric symptoms may be referred to as having "Silent" or "Inobvious" Strokes.

Peter Birkett, MD, is Associate Research Scientist in the Department of Psychiatry, at Columbia University Center for Geriatrics and Gerontology, and on the Faculty of Medicine at Columbia University. He also is currently serving as Medical Director at the Riverside Nursing Home, in Haverstraw, NY.

[Haworth co-indexing entry note]: "The Psychiatry of Stroke." Birkett, D. Peter. Co-published simultaneously in *Loss, Grief & Care* (The Haworth Press, Inc.) Vol. 8, No. 1/2, 1998, pp. 15-22; and: *After Stroke: Enhancing Quality of Life* (ed: Wallace Sife) The Haworth Press, Inc., 1998, pp. 15-22. Single or multiple copies of this article are available for a fee from The Haworth Document Delivery Service [1-800-342-9678, 9:00 a.m. - 5:00 p.m. (EST). E-mail address: getinfo@haworth.com].

STROKE RISK FACTORS

Psychiatry is involved in the stroke risk factors because some stroke risk factors, such as cocaine use, produce behavioral problems. Others, such as smoking and non-adherence to hypertension treatment, require behavioral management. Personality factors leading to stroke have not been well established, but repressed anger and the "Type A" personality are current focuses of research. This area of prevention overlaps with treatment, because prevention of a second stroke is an important part of stroke treatment.

ANATOMY AND BIOCHEMISTRY

The relationship between the site of the infarct and mental symptoms caused is of theoretical, as well as practical, interest. Patients with right-sided infarcts are generally more likely to have behavioral disturbances than are those with right hemiplegia. This may be a result of the greater neurological disability associated with left infarcts, which overshadows mental disabilities.

Strategically located infarcts may affect particular neurotransmitters. The main neurotransmitter-producing areas for catecholamines are in the locus ceruieus, for acetylcholine in the nucleus of Meyneit, for serotonin in the raphe (midline) gray matter in the pons and medulla, and for dopamine in the substantia nigra. It is thus possible that strokes affecting these areas are especially likely to cause defects in certain neurotransmitters.

COMMUNICATION DISORDERS

Speech disorders interact with psychiatric disorders to such an extent that complete distinction may not be possible. In expressive aphasias the limitation of the disability to speech, rather than to other aspects of memory and intellect, can be detected. Receptive aphasias can result in unintelligible speech resembling that of psychosis or dementia. Receptive and global aphasias may mimic dementia but there is preservation of the capacity for complex behavior skills, although these may be impaired by neurological defects.

HALLUCINATIONS AND VISUAL DISORDERS

Auditory hallucinations are rare in stroke but several kinds of visual disturbances may occur. The distinction between neurological and psychiatric causes of visual disturbance may be incomplete or impossible, especially in the presence of dementia. Exact diagnosis and explanation of a neuro-ophthalmic disorder may be therapeutic. In some cases the patient may resent having the disability pointed out. Cases with occipital infarcts may mimic "hysterical" blindness and need the same kind of management. Agnosias may respond to reeducation and training, and some cases may need treatment for depression. Hallucinations tend to occur in the blind areas of visual field defects. Hallucinations are so common and due to so many causes that the presence of an infarct should not prevent a search for other treatable causes, including delirium and psychosis.

DISORDERS OF SOMATIC SENSATION

Parietal lobe syndromes are due to disturbances in awareness of body sensation. They include apraxia and some kinds of anosognosia. These syndromes may overlap, or be confused with, dementia and emotional disorders. Loss of sensation is difficult to detect if communication is limited, and can lead to difficulties in rehabilitation.

Pain in stroke has several psychiatric implications. The thalamic pain syndrome, consisting of spontaneous pain on the affected side, following a stroke with mild hemiplegia, sometimes responds better to anti-depressant medications than to analgesics. Sub-arachnoid hemorrhage often presents as a severe headache and negative doctor-patient relationships can delay the correct diagnosis.

SEX

The emotional effects of stroke, together with such factors as blood pressure medications, diabetes, and vascular disease, may reduce sexual activity. Vascular disease may affect the penile arteries. In vasculogenic impotence sexual fantasy and desire persist but there is loss of capacity for erection. Orgasm in female stroke victims is frequently lost. Most stroke occurs in the elderly, and this affects expectations of sexual function.

APATHY AND FAILURE OF REHABILITATION

Upper motor neuron paralysis is less complete than lower motor neuron paralysis, and return of mobility can be influenced by motivation. It is possible that certain lesions in the frontal lobe, caudate nucleus and thalamus specifically cause apathy. Cognitive impairment also impairs stroke rehabilitation. In older patients it can be hard to tell whether they have resumed normal social roles because social roles are less clearly defined in later life. There is a direct effect of stroke in producing fatigue. Medical disorders can be misinterpreted as psychological apathy in stroke. Potentially sedative medications given to stroke patients include psychotropics, hypnotics, benzodiazepines, anticonvulsants and beta blockers. Valuable clues may come from conversations with the family or care givers.

Social circumstances and mental state, especially dementia, are stronger predictors of recovery of function than is the medical condition. Age is the most consistent predictor. Social isolation carries a high risk for poor outcome.

Patients want to see a direct connection between rehabilitation methods and their expected goals. Young patients are often intolerant of rehabilitation procedures that they cannot perceive as immediately leading to desired objectives. The benefits of rehabilitation treatment beyond the acute phase have been questioned because it often cannot be shown objectively to improve physical recovery. But its effects on emotional well-being and morale are not to be ignored.

ANGER

Outbursts of apparent anger are common in stroke, but we cannot always be sure of the precise emotion felt. Many medications have been used in treatment of violent behavior, but the results have been equivocal and they may be acting as chemical straitjackets or non-specific sedatives rather than reducing angry feelings. Sedation risks are enhanced in the stroke patient by the frequent presence of cardiovascular disease. Other treatment measures include reassurance of the caregivers, placement in the correct setting, management on a psychiatric unit in a general hospital, providing space, avoiding unnecessary physical contacts, a patient advocate, and an interdisciplinary care plan. In formulating the care plan it is useful to identify the target behavior, measure its frequency, observe what precipitates it, and identify the victims. It may be necessary to modify medical treatment regimes and to tolerate non-violent disturbances of behavior.

DISINHIBITION

Stroke can cause weakening of normal social constraints on behavior. Management must address the concerns of those affected by the behavior, as well as the patient. Aberrant actions can result from cognitive impairment in dementia and delirium. In some cases of frontal lobe syndrome there is euphoria and disinhibition. Frontal lobe damage is often due to sub-arachnoid hemorrhage from a ruptured congenital aneurysm.

PARANOIA

Delusions in organic disorder are commonly accompanied by confusion, but also have certain distinctive features apart from this. Misidentification syndromes, such as delusions that family members have been replaced by imposters, may be due to either functional psychosis or to organic brain damage, most commonly right-sided infarcts. The location of the lesion has not been consistently shown to have a major effect on the presence or absence of delusions, but the right hemisphere in general, posterior areas in general, and the left temporal lobe have been suggested as more likely locations. Patients may need care in a protected setting but inappropriate placement is common. Anti-psychotic medication is useful but very paranoid patients may refuse it, and side-effects of drowsiness and parkinsonism may be especially difficult in stroke.

DEPRESSION

There is evidence for an entity of "post-stroke depression" which has certain specific features, and is not merely a reaction to a depressing situation. This may depend on the location of the infarct, and there is evidence that it is especially associated with left anterior infarcts. Other negative moods, such as anxiety and irritability, may mimic depression in stroke. Spontaneous weeping in stroke may cause distress, but is not due to major depression.

Stroke patients themselves attach more importance to friendly and encouraging attitudes than to specific anti-depressant treatments such as medications. Social work services to help with finances and housing and social isolation are often needed. Anti-depressant drugs may have cardiovascular or epileptogenic side-effects that are significant in stroke. Some cases of depression respond better to ECT than to drugs or psychotherapy. ECT causes a slight transient rise in blood pressure, but has been used safely in stroke, and the main risks are those of anesthesia.

ANXIETY

Panic attacks and agoraphobia do not typically precede stroke, and stroke does not come at the culmination of anything subjectively resembling anxiety. The emotional reaction on return to consciousness after stroke is bewildered and dream-like, but is not typically dominated by fear. Subsequent to recovery, fear of a second stroke becomes prominent. Anxiety and nervousness are more frequent in the first year after the stroke, but thereafter tend to improve. Treatments for anxiety include medication and psychotherapy. Most drugs which reduce anxiety can cause drowsiness, probably due to a common site of action at the $GABA_a$ receptor, and this is a problem when using them in stroke. Explanation and reassurance about the illness are especially important in anxiety, following stroke.

DEMENTIA

Most demented patients who do not have severe Alzheimer's disease are found at autopsy or on CAT scan to have brain infarcts. The overlap between Alzheimer's disease and vascular dementia is probably no more or less than due to chance. The consensus of the literature is that vascular dementia is less common than Alzheimer's disease. A history of stroke or the presence of an infarct on CAT scan are commonly used to distinguish vascular dementia from Alzheimer's disease. The onset of illness is often more sudden in vascular dementia, and there are more episodes of sudden deterioration.

Multiplicity of the infarcts is commonly regarded as a factor in causing dementia. The presence of dementia may also be related to having infarcts in both the thalamus and the cortex, and to their being bilateral. Infarcts with a volume of less than 100 ml are unlikely to cause dementia. Infarcts of the frontal lobes and the hippocampus are commoner in the demented than the nondemented.

Helping caregivers with social and economic problems is probably more important than any specific treatment. Vascular dementia may be reduced by controlling high blood pressure, but it is important to avoid episodes of hypotension. Exercise, aspirin, and giving up smoking have been claimed to help. Anti-psychotic medications are used in treatment of the behavioral complications of dementia. Reality orientation is used to improve awareness, but is not of proven effectiveness.

PSYCHOTHERAPY

Emotional well-being and morale may be helped by psychotherapy, but psychotherapists have difficulties in dealing with the brain-damaged. Psychotherapy with stroke patients is often impeded by dementia or aphasia. The dynamic aspects of therapy often concern the relationship between the patients and the care givers. Direct advice and counseling are often needed, and knowledge of entitlements to Medicaid and Medicare and Social Security and disability benefits can be more useful to the patient than technical medical or psychiatric expertise. Support groups of various kinds can be helpful, and information can be provided by organizations such as the National Stroke Association.

CAREGIVERS

The mental effects of stroke cause more stress than the physical, for family care givers. Family care givers suffer sleep problems, social isolation, and financial burdens, and report feeling anxiety and depression. The problems families encounter with health and social agencies may need advocate services, rather than mental health services.

Professionals who help care for stroke often suffer emotional strain. The team approach can reduce such strain, as well as facilitate the formation and documentation of treatment plans.

WHERE SHOULD THE STROKE PATIENT BE TREATED AND BY WHOM?

It is medically recommended that all stroke victims should be hospitalized, but this is not always done. Psycho-social factors probably predominate in the decision. Most hospital-treated stroke patients go back to their own homes, and most of the rest to nursing homes. OBRA'87 (the Omnibus Reconciliation Act of 1987) was intended to stop the mentally ill from being put in nursing homes, but made an exemption for dementia. The "loophole" has resulted in nursing homes continuing to hold many stroke victims with mental illness.

The basic problem is that stroke is not an illness that fits our present categories. The stroke patient suffers multiple handicaps that cut across disciplinary boundaries and render imperative the need for the inter-disciplinary team approach. No stroke problems are simple or isolated, and they are not restricted solely to the survivor of a stroke.

This need for inter-disciplinary team approach was brought to me poignantly. A member of the audience at one of these meetings approached Dr. Kutscher and me to tell the story of how her father had suffered a stroke and was refused admission to a general hospital because his problems were behavioral. He was then refused admission to a psychiatric unit, on the grounds that stroke was not a mental illness, and he was put in a nursing home. He walked out, went back home, and killed her mother.

Focused Stroke Rehabilitation Programs:
A Review of Prospective Controlled Trials

Michael J. Reding

Major advances have been made in the medical and surgical management of stroke. Through carefully designed controlled studies we now have firm data to support the use of aspirin for prevention of further TIA or stroke due to platelet thromboemboli, the use of Coumadin® to prevent cardiac embolic strokes due to atrial fibrillation, and the use of carotid endarterectomy for treatment of symptomatic carotid artery stenosis. Equally compelling data support the role of focused stroke rehabilitation teams in the management of functional disabilities following stroke.

Prospective randomized studies currently available in the world literature allow us to make several affirmations concerning the value of stroke rehabilitation. They will be discussed in turn as follows: (1) Rehabilitation has a differential effect on self-care functional deficits as opposed to neurologic impairments. (2) The more focused the rehabilitation program the better the outcome. (3) No one rehabilitation approach has been shown to be better than any other. (4) Cost effective use of rehabilitation resources requires selection of patients most likely to benefit.

REHABILITATION AFFECTS DISABILITY MORE THAN IMPAIRMENT

The value of stroke rehabilitation is usually discussed in terms of its effect on recovery of ambulation and self-care function. It is important to

Michael J. Reding, MD, is Associate Professor of Neurology, Cornell University Medical College, and Director of Stroke Rehabilitation at Burke Rehabilitation Hospital in White Plains, NY. Dr. Reding is Board certified in internal medicine and neurology.

[Haworth co-indexing entry note]: "Focused Stroke Rehabilitation Programs: A Review of Prospective Controlled Trials." Reding, Michael J. Co-published simultaneously in Loss, Grief & Care (The Haworth Press, Inc.) Vol. 8, No. 1/2, 1998, pp. 23-36; and: After Stroke: Enhancing Quality of Life (ed: Wallace Sife) The Haworth Press, Inc., 1998, pp. 23-36. Single or multiple copies of this article are available for a fee from The Haworth Document Delivery Service [1-800-342-9678, 9:00 a.m. - 5:00 p.m. (EST). E-mail address: getinfo@haworth.com].

review our use of the term "function" as opposed to "impairment." The World Health Organization has emphasized that neurologic injury is manifested at different levels as: pathology, neurologic impairment, functional disability and handicap.[1] Pathology is expressed as a structural abnormality at the tissue level. The effect of stroke on brain function produces a neurologic impairment: hemiparesis, hemihypesthesia, ataxia. Stroke at the level of the organism as a whole produces a disability, interfering with the way individuals walk, dress, and care for themselves. The next level of effect of a stroke on the individual is called handicap. Handicap is the effect of stroke on the individual's ability to function within the family, socially, and at work.

One does not expect rehabilitation to affect pathology, the encephalomalacic area within the brain. It is uncertain whether rehabilitation affects the neurologic impairments: weakness, sensory loss, hemianoptic visual deficit, etc.

Rehabilitation has been shown to minimize disability by enhancing self-care function. If a patient is weak and has trouble walking then a cane and brace may be helpful. If a patient is hemiparetic and has trouble dressing then adapted clothing, changing clothing styles, or using hemiplegic dressing techniques may be helpful. Rehabilitation after stroke teaches patients to use devices and techniques which improve their ability to perform self-care functional activities appropriate for their spectrum and severity of neurologic impairments.

Rehabilitation devices and training are also helpful in minimizing the effects of stroke on the patient's handicap interacting with others socially and in the workplace. Home and work modifications, for example, allow wheelchair accessibility to bathroom, recreational, and work facilities and enable patients to remain productive family and community members.

VALUE OF REHABILITATION: RANDOMIZED TRIALS

It is important to realize that rehabilitation is provided in different settings and at different intensities. The inpatient rehabilitation experience is most intense with 24 hour medical and nursing rehabilitation care, plus rehabilitation therapy sessions 5 days per week. It implies that the patient has more need for assistance with ADL function, has perhaps more intensive nursing care needs, feeding tubes, bladder care, catheterization and need for medical supervision. Outpatient rehabilitation is usually recommended if the patient can be easily mobilized in the community and get from home to the outpatient clinic with reasonable effort. The next level of rehabilitation care is homecare with the therapist treating the patient at home. This is the rehabilitation option of choice if the patient is functionally able to be discharged home but is not able to be brought into the outpatient clinic for logistical reasons.

Rehabilitation is a process which occurs over time. The acute phase of rehabilitation is usually described as the first two weeks after stroke. The subacute phase is from two weeks to six months. The chronic phase begins 6 months after stroke. There is an exponential recovery curve during the acute and subacute phase. Progress is still seen during the chronic phase but the rate of change is much slower.

With the above issues in mind, it is apparent that there are a number of factors to be considered in studying the value of rehabilitation following stroke. Studies should be designed using a prospective randomization technique with use of a control group to evaluate the effects of spontaneous recovery on rehabilitation outcome. To be relevant, studies should assess the effects of rehabilitation on disability, not neurologic impairment. The intensity of rehabilitation, the setting in which it was delivered, and the time interval following stroke at which patients were treated should all be specified.

A literature review shows that there are no prospective studies which compare patients not receiving rehabilitation therapy with those enrolled in a rehabilitation program. Such a study is usually considered unethical as it would deprive patients of treatment which is considered usual and customary. There are 5 studies which randomize patients to alternate rehabilitation care on a general medical unit versus rehabilitation on a focused stroke rehabilitation unit (see Table 1). Patients on the medical ward received physical, occupational, and speech therapy, but the process was not part of a focused team approach to the patient's functional, and social support needs. The randomization process in these studies is usually based upon which service had a bed available.

The first such study was in 1979 by Feigenson et al.[2] Patients were randomized on admission to a rehabilitation hospital to go either to a general rehabilitation ward or to a focused stroke rehabilitation ward. The authors looked at functional outcome for the two patient groups. Both groups received rehabilitation services. On the general rehabilitation ward the therapists and nursing staff dealt with the full gamut of rehabilitation problems: stroke, head injury, multiple sclerosis, Guillian Barré Syndrome, orthopedic rehabilitation, amputation, etc. The stroke unit admitted only patients with stroke. Over 600 patients were studied. There was significant benefit in favor of the stroke unit with better ambulation scores and fewer patients requiring nursing home placement.

The next study was published in 1980 by Gaff et al. from Edinburgh,

TABLE 1. Focused Stroke Rehabilitation Improves Function
(Randomized Controlled Trials)

REFERENCE		SIZE	BENEFIT
FEIGENSON,	Stroke 1979; 10:5-8	n = 667	Ambulation Home Discharge
GARRAWAY,	Br. Med. J. 1980; 280:1040-1043	n = 307	Ambulation Self-Care
SMITH,*	Br. Med. J. 1981; 282:517-520	n = 133*	Ambulation Self-Care
STRAND,	Stroke, 1985; 16:29-34	n = 293	Ambulation Self-Care Length of Stay
KASTE,	World Stroke Cong. 1992; S27	n = 243	Self-Care Length of Stay Home Discharge

* Outpatient Program 4 days/week at 6 hrs/day vs. 3 days/week for 3 hrs/day vs. home care, no rehabilitation

Scotland.[3] This again was a situationally randomized study. Patients were randomized from the emergency room to go either to a stroke unit or to a general medical ward. On the stroke unit the physician, physical therapy, occupational therapy, speech therapy, social work, and nursing staff all worked as a team. They met regularly to discuss patient goals, progress, and problems. They had protocols in place to assess and treat the medical and rehabilitation problems frequently encountered in patients following stroke. On the general medical ward every patient received rehabilitation services but they were not part of a coordinated team approach. The study consisted of 370 patients. There were statistically significant improvements noted in favor of the stroke unit in ambulation scores and also in self-care scores.

Smith et al. from Northwick Hospital outside of London randomized 133 patients in the emergency room to be admitted either to a general medical ward or to a stroke unit.[4] They found significantly greater improvements in ambulation and self-care scores in favor of the stroke unit.

Strand et al. in a study from Sweden randomized 293 patients seen in the emergency room to be admitted to a general medical ward or to a stroke ward based upon bed availability.[5] They found significant benefits in favor of the stroke unit for ambulation scores, self-care scores, and length-of-stay.

Another study by Kaste et al. from Finland with a similar design and a sample size of 243 found benefit in favor of the stroke unit for self-care scores, length-of-stay and need for nursing home placements.

These studies are best summarized by saying that there is now an international consensus that focused stroke rehabilitation units improve ambulation scores, self-care scores and need for nursing home placement for patients with stroke.

There was a study by Wade et al. in 1985 that studied the effects of patient randomization to stroke rehabilitation at home versus nursing visits to the home with appropriate health and hygiene recommendations.[7] They studied 800 patients. Those randomized to receive home rehabilitation care were seen by a physical therapist, an occupational therapist, and a speech therapist. The therapists were working a half-day schedule and evaluated and treated 400 patients over two years. Working five half-days per week each therapist had to evaluate four new patients a week, in addition to treating those receiving ongoing therapy. They found no beneficial effects of the home rehabilitation program. Their study design has been criticized for its lack of intensity. There are many other possible reasons why they failed to demonstrate a treatment effect. Such negative studies are of limited value, especially when positive effects have been demonstrated by five different research groups as cited above.

NO ONE REHABILITATION PHILOSOPHY HAS BEEN SHOWN TO BE SUPERIOR TO OTHERS

It is not clear what is the optimal rehabilitation treatment approach. There are two divergent philosophical approaches; one tries to restore normal or near normal movement, and the other tries to substitute for the loss of movement by using preserved muscle groups. The following authors have written therapy texts which aim to restore normal movement. In 1956 Knott and Voss published the Proprioceptive Neuromuscular Facilitation (PNF).[8] In 1972 the Bobaths published the Neurodevelopmental Technique (NDT)[9]. Karr and Shepherd developed the Motor Relearning Program (MRP) which was published in 1985.[10] The traditional approach allows–even encourages–the substitution of preserved functions for those which have been lost.[11] The main treatment goal is functional movement. Quality of movement is of secondary importance. The Brunnstrom approach uses spinal cord segmental and supra segmental reflexes to facilitate movement. [12] Rehabilitation techniques for treatment of hemiparesis following stroke can thus be quite contradictory in their approaches. There are several prospectively randomized controlled studies which examine differences in outcome for patients treated according to one philosophy versus another (see Table 2).

In 1970 Stem et al. studied the effect of the PNF as described by Knott and Voss versus "traditional therapy."[13] They defined traditional therapy as a functionally oriented approach to improve self care and ambulation using whatever substitution techniques, walking assist devices or bracing needed to improve self-care and ambulation function. They used the Kenny self-care and ambulation scale to measure outcome. There was no difference in outcome for the two treatment groups. All patients improved.

Loggigian et al. have conducted a similar study comparing outcome for patients treated using neurodevelopmental techniques versus traditional therapy.[14] With a sample size of 42 patients they found no differential benefit of one treatment approach versus the other.

Dickstein et al. studied patients treated by one of three approaches: PNF, NDT or traditional therapy.[15] Each of the 3 treatment groups had approximately 40 patients. They found no preferential benefit for PNF versus NDT versus traditional therapy.

Wagenaar et al. studied seven patients using an "A-B-A" design comparing the outcome for patients treated using NDT versus Brunnstrom treatment techniques.[16] Outcome scores measuring ADL function, strength, and quality of movement were similar for all three treatment approaches.

TABLE 2. Physical Therapy Techniques Equally Effective

REFERENCE		SIZE	TECHNIQUES COMPARED
STERN,	Arch. Phys. Med. Rehabil. 1970; 71; 526-531	n = 62	PNF vs. Traditional
LOGGIGAN,	Arch. Phys. Med. 1983; 64:634-637	n = 42	NDT vs. Traditional
DICKSTEIN	Phys. Ther. 1986; 66:1233-1238	n = 131	PNF vs. NDT vs. Traditional
WAGENAAR,	Scand. J. Rehab. Med. 1990; 22:1-8	n = 7	NDT vs. Brunnstrom
SALTER,	Rehab. Nursing 1991; 16:62-66	n = 80	NDT vs. Traditional

Salter et al. set up a NDT rehabilitation team on one stroke rehabilitation unit.[17] On another stroke rehabilitation ward they continued using traditional therapy. They found no differential benefit in favor of either unit.

The above studies comparing alternate rehabilitation treatment strategies can be summarized by saying that at the present time no one therapy approach is better than any other. Decisions concerning which techniques to use should be left to the judgment and experience of the treating therapist.

REHABILITATION SELECTION CRITERIA

All patients with stroke are not the same. The location, size, and number of strokes differ from one patient to another. They are obviously not expected to recover in a uniform pattern. Patients with a pure motor hemiparesis have the best prognosis. Those with hemiparesis and hemihypesthesia show an intermediate rate of recovery. Those with hemiparesis, hemihypesthesia, and hemianoptic visual deficits show the slowest and most incomplete recovery. Figure 1 shows the probability of being able to walk 150 feet without assistance for patients with different combinations of motor, somatic sensory, and hemianoptic visual deficits.[18,19] There is a ninety-five percent probability that patients with pure motor hemiparesis will be able to walk independently by about 14 weeks post stroke. Patients with hemihypesthesia and motor weakness have a 40 percent probability of walking independently by about 18 weeks following stroke. Patients with hemiparesis, hemihypesthesia, and hemianoptic visual deficits are unlikely to walk independently during the first 30 weeks post stroke. This does not mean that they are inappropriate for rehabilitation. Their goals are different. They are expected to be able to walk with assistance. Such a goal allows for assisted ambulation within the home with the patient able to walk from room to room.

Figure 2 is a life table plot showing the probability of reaching a Barthel score of 95 or greater indicating independence with feeding, dressing, grooming, bathing, toileting, ambulation, and stair climbing for patients with different neurologic impairments.[18,19] Comparing Figures 1 and 2 shows that patients with pure motor hemiparesis are likely to be independent with walking, but only 75 percent will be independent with self-care. Figure 3 shows that even for the patient population with hemiparesis, hemihypesthesia, and hemianoptic visual deficits there is a fifty percent probability of reaching a Barthel score of 60. This represents a functional level at which point home care becomes more efficient.[20] An aged spouse

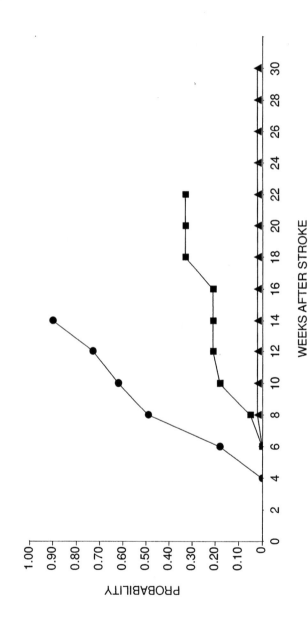

FIGURE 1. Probability of Walking ≥ 150 ft. Without Assistance

LIFE TABLE ANALYSIS

MOTOR DEFICIT
MOTOR, SENSORY DEFICIT
MOTOR, SENSORY, VISUAL DEFICIT

30

can assist such patients with their ADL activities, with walking and with transfers.

The goal of rehabilitation following stroke is to maximize ADL and mobility function, and return the patient to the community as independent as possible. Patients with pure motor hemiparesis are expected to reach independence with ADL and mobility function. These goals are likely to be achieved irrespective of support by available family members. For patients with more extensive neurologic impairments the probability of their reaching independence with self care and ambulation is lower. The goal of returning the patient to the community will depend upon the availability of supervision and assistance in the home. If one judges the value of rehabilitation by assessing the number of patients requiring nursing home placement then the assessment will be clouded by social issues beyond the reach of rehabilitation staff. Even the most skilled rehabilitation staff can not provide a spouse or other interested family member to assist the patient with their home care. If the value of rehabilitation is judged by discharge disposition then selection criteria for rehabilitation must consider both the severity of the patient's stroke and the availability of family or community support.

Figure 3 shows that the rehabilitation process doesn't just produce a transient effect.[21] This figure shows the results of 2 year follow-up phone interviews with patients or their caregiver following discharge from the inpatient stroke rehabilitation unit at Burke Rehabilitation Hospital. The mean admission Barthel score was 30. The mean Barthel score at the time of discharge from the inpatient stroke unit was 60. There was a slight decline in Barthel scores over the subsequent 2 year follow-up interval, but the decline was not statistically significant. The value of the rehabilitation process thus seems to be durable, persisting over 2 years following discharge from the inpatient unit.

There is a general consensus that the older the patient the worse the rehabilitation outcome.[22] This is probably true for unselected patients since the older the person is, the more likely they are to have functionally significant comorbidity: dementia, obstructive pulmonary disease, congestive heart failure, angina pectoris, degenerative arthritic problems, etc. It is easy to exclude such overriding comorbid problems by selecting only those patients who were independent in the community before their stroke. If they had the cognitive, cardiopulmonary and musculoskeletal capacity to function independently outside their homes within the community then their functional outcome is not significantly different than that observed for their younger colleagues. Older patients also have more advanced atherosclerosis with poorer collateral flow and larger infarcts compared to

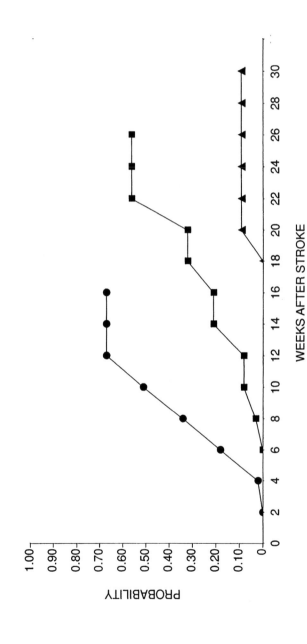

FIGURE 2. Probability of Reaching a Barthel Score ≥ 95

LIFE TABLE ANALYSIS

MOTOR DEFICIT ●●
MOTOR, SENSORY DEFICIT ■■
MOTOR, SENSORY, VISUAL DEFICIT ▲▲

32

FIGURE 3. Mean Barthel Index Score versus Time

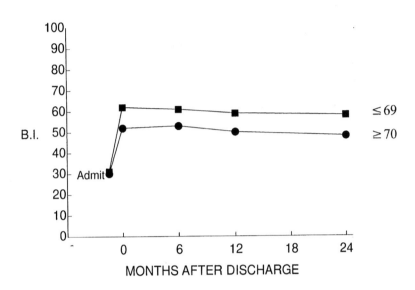

their younger colleagues. To correct for this, comparisons of outcome for older versus younger stroke patients should be matched for severity of stroke related neurologic impairments. This is shown in Figure 4, a life-table plot of the probability of walking 150 ft. without assistance for older versus younger patients with pure motor paresis selected for rehabilitation using the above mentioned selection criteria.

In summary, the literature reviewed above supports the value of focused stroke rehabilitation units. There is no clear advantage of one rehabilitation treatment approach versus another. Selection criteria for rehabilitation hospital admission can be used to select patients most likely to benefit. Life-table outcome plots can be used to define the probability of reaching ADL and ambulation goals, and estimate the time required to reach these goals. Discharge to home versus to a nursing home depends upon the type and severity of the patient's neurologic impairments, and availability of family support.

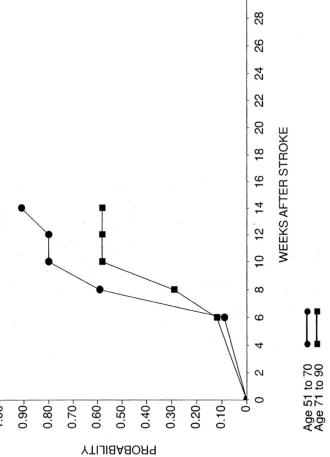

FIGURE 4. Probability of Walking ≥ 150 ft. Without Assistance
Motor Deficit Only

WEEKS AFTER STROKE

PROBABILITY

Age 51 to 70
Age 71 to 90

BIBLIOGRAPHY

1. World Health Organization: International Classification of Impairments, Disabilities, and Handicaps: A Manual of Classification Relating to the Consequences of Disease. Geneva, World Health Organization, 1980.

2. Feigenson J., Gitlow H., Greenberg D. The disability oriented stroke unit: A major factor influencing stroke outcome. Stroke 1979; 10:5-8.

3. Garraway W., Akhtar A., Prescott R., Hockey L. Management of Acute Stroke in the Elderly: Preliminary Results of a Controlled Trial. Br Med J 1980; 280:1040-1043.

4. Smith D., Goldenberg E., Ashbum A., Kinsella G., Sheikh K. et al. Remedial therapy after stroke: A randomised controlled trial. Br Med Jour. 1981; 282:517-520.

5. Strand T., Asplund K., Eriksson S., Hagg E., Lithner F., Wester P. A nonintensive stroke unit reduces functional disability and the need for long-term hospitalization. Stroke 1985; 16:29-34.

6. Kaste M., Palomaki H. Who should treat elderly stroke patients? Presented at The Second World Congress of Stroke, 1992, Washington DC, Sept. 8-12, page 527, National Stroke Assn. Publ., Englewood Colorado, 1992.

7. Wade D., Langton-Hewer R., Skilbeck C., Bainton D., Burns-Cox C. Controlled Trial of a Home-Care Service for Acute Stroke Patients. Lancet 1985; Feb 9: 323-326.

8. Knott M., Voss D. Proprioceptive Neuromuscular Facilitation: Patterns and Techniques. Harper & Row, New York 1956.

9. Bobath B. Adult Hemiplegia: Evaluation and Treatment. William Heinemann Medical Books, London 1970.

10. Carr, J. & Shepherd, R. A Motor Relearning Programme for Stroke. William Heinemann Medical Books, London, 1983.

11. Price S., Reding M. Physical Therapy Philosophies and Strategies. In *Handbook of Neurorehabilitation*. Good D, and Couch J., editors. Marcel Dekker Publ., New York 1994.

12. Brunnstrom S. Movement Therapy in Hemiplegia: A Neurophysiological Approach. Harper & Row, Philadelphia 1970.

13. Stern H., McDowell F., Miller J., Robinson M. Arch Phys Med Rehabil 1970; 51: 526-531.

14. Loggigian M., Samuels M., Falconer J. et al. Clinical exercise trial for stroke patients. Arch Phys Med Rehabil 1983; 64: 364-367.

15. Dickstein R., Hocherman S., Pillar T., Shaham R. Phys Ther 1986; 66: 1233-1238.

16. Wagenaar R., Meijer, O., Van Wieringen P., Kuik D., Hazenberg G. et al. Scand. J. Rehabil Med 1990; 22: 1-8.

17. Salter J., Camp Y., Pierce L., Mion L. Rehabilitation Nursing Approaches to Cerebrovascular Accident: A Comparison of two Approaches. Rehabilitation Nursing 1991; 16: 62-66.

18. Reding M., Potes E. Rehabilitation outcome following initial unilateral hemispheric stroke: A life table analysis approach. Stroke 1988; 19: 1354-1358.

19. Reding M. A model stroke classification scheme and its use in outcome research. Stroke 1990; 21(Suppl 2): 35-37.

20. Granger C., Dewis L, Peters N., Sherwood C., Barrett J. Stroke Rehabilitation: Analysis and Repeated Barthel Index Scores. Arch Phys Med Rehabil 1979; 60: 14-17.

21. Borucki S., Volpe B, Reding M. The effect of age on maintenance of functional gains following stroke rehabilitation. J Neuro Rehab 1992; 6: 1-5.

22. Reding M. Age and its Effect on Rehabilitation Outcome Following Stroke. In *Practicing Rehabilitation With Geriatric Clients*. Dermot-Frengley J., Murray P., Wykle M., editors. Springer Publ Co., New York, 1990.

Psychological Studies
in Stroke Rehabilitation

Leonard Diller
Dvorah Simon

Many years ago my colleagues and I were struck by the fact that there were significant developments in the field of neuropsychology, which increased our understanding of brain behavior relationships. There were also important developments in stroke rehabilitation, in improving procedures and outcomes. However, the two lines of knowledge and experiences were not in communication with each other. For example, what was one to do with a psychological test protocol which indicated that a person could not copy a figure correctly or respond to a simple reasoning problem? The question of the presence and even the locus and extent of brain damage was basically secondary to the reason why the person was being referred. We knew that the individual was brain damaged, otherwise he would not be there. From a rehabilitation perspective there was a question of what to do with the data. We concluded that neuropsychologists stopped thinking when rehabilitation started. We also determined that rehabilita-

---

Leonard Diller, PhD, is Director of Psychology at Rusk Institute of Rehabilitation Medicine, and Professor of Clinical Rehabilitation Medicine, NYU School of Medicine. He has served as President of the American Congress of Rehabilitation Medicine, Division of Psychology, APA, and is the author of more than 100 articles and chapters. Dvorah Simon, PhD, is a psychologist at Rusk Institute Rehabilitation Medicine, and Assistant Clinical Professor of Rehabilitation Medicine at NYU School of Medicine. She has been involved in federally funded psychological research into aspects of rehabilitation from CVA and traumatic brain injury, and is actively presenting on these subjects.

[Haworth co-indexing entry note]: "Psychological Studies in Stroke Rehabilitation." Diller, Leonard, and Dvorah Simon. Co-published simultaneously in *Loss, Grief & Care* (The Haworth Press, Inc.) Vol. 8, No. 1/2, 1998, pp. 37-43; and: *After Stroke: Enhancing Quality of Life* (ed: Wallace Sife) The Haworth Press, Inc., 1998, pp. 37-43. Single or multiple copies of this article are available for a fee from The Haworth Document Delivery Service [1-800-342-9678, 9:00 a.m. - 5:00 p.m. (EST). E-mail address: getinfo@haworth.com].

37

tion workers lacked a rationale for systematic procedures because of an emphasis on functional results and resolution of multiproblem circumstances, glossing over details of impairments.

A rehabilitation center is basically a school for teaching people how to adapt to or overcome impairments and disabilities. Rehabilitation can be pictured as a variant or extension of special education, where people go to class to acquire skills. Special education began at the turn of the 18th century, with physicians who were applying the neurophysiology of their time, to problems of children who were raised in the wild, or were deaf or delayed in learning. The field was originated and invigorated by physicians from Itard to Montessori, and was then left to the teaching profession. Looking at a rehabilitation center as a school, we note people are eligible if they have disabilities based on impairments, and can benefit from three hours a day of daily instruction, in classes conducted by PTs, OTs and speech therapists. This special education metaphor was useful in several ways.

I was asked by our speech department to examine a patient, who was described as depressed, severely aphasic, and silent during speech therapy sessions. On psychological examination, I concluded that the patient was indeed depressed, aphasic, and did not speak. Not knowing what to do with this redundant information, I observed a speech therapy session through a one way mirror. But, looking through such a mirror I realized that I had no tools or parameters to define what I was looking for. For want of anything better, I took a stop watch and timed who was talking at each 10 second interval. When I counted the intervals over a half hour period, I realized that I had recorded 180 observational trials, and found that the therapist talked during 50 per cent of these trials, and the patient less than 10 per cent. The rest was silence. I had found a way of framing the therapist's referral into metrics which could suggest paths for intervention. Similarly, in observing patients with "perceptual problems" in occupational therapy, one noticed that when the therapist was presenting a stimulus, the patient was looking at the face of the therapist for approval, rather than at the stimuli or the task procedures. My colleague, Joseph Weinberg, and I concluded that a major deficit in patients was a difficulty in paying attention to what was being taught. From the perspective of teaching/learning, attention seemed to be a critical starting point to look at the interplay of neuropsychological and rehabilitation phenomena.

To get a systematic look at attention, we devised a small test battery, taking into account that left hemisphere patients, who were largely aphasic, might have problems in processing auditory information, while right hemispheric damaged patients might have more difficulty in processing spatial information. We made a distinction between the kind of attention involved in searching the environment, versus the attention required in maintaining or holding on to information. We devised a brief test battery based on these ideas, consisting of a search test in which the individual had to scan the environment for targets, and a test in which the individual had to retain information. The former we called scan, the latter we called span. We presented each of these through visual as well as auditory modalities. For scanning we devised a simple cancellation test, requiring the individual to cross out a target in a visual display or to raise his/her hand when the correct target was read aloud in a series of targets. For span, we took a digit span test commonly used as part of intelligence tests and made a visual analogue where the subject was shown a series of numbers and then had to point out the correct sequence when the series was removed.

The results were interesting. Individuals with left hemisphere damage did poorly on the auditory scan and span tests. They did well on visual scan tests in terms of not having many errors, but their responses were very slow. Responses to visual span were mixed. We thought that despite the visual nature of the task demands, it had serial components which relate to maintaining information over time. Right hemisphere damaged patients did poorly on visual scan (cancellation) and to a lesser extent on visual span. Visual cancellation responses were characterized by many errors of omission. There were no errors of commission, e.g., canceling the wrong targets. There were far more errors on the side of the page opposite the lesion. Finally there was great variability. We could divide the patients into three groups: those with many errors, those with few errors, and those in the middle. Patients with many errors and some in the middle group tended to exhibit many different ways of going about the task. Some would start from left to right. Some would go up and down. Some would seem to go in a random catch as catch can way (Diller et al., 1974).

A most interesting finding was that right hemisphere-damaged patients generally did well on auditory tests, both on auditory cancellation as well as digit span forwards. However, digit span backwards was a problem. While most normal people are slightly better on digits forward than digits backward, these patients were decidedly inferior. We were puzzled by this finding, which has since been confirmed by others. Although it can be understood as a difficulty in holding onto information while processing it for retrieval, we also suggest that the visual system is involved in processing this kind of information. Phenomenologically, there is an eye movement. One can test this by spelling one's own name backwards and noticing how the letters appear to be stored and read off.

Our findings lead us to examine in several ways, attentional difficulties in right brain damaged people. We examined the clinical correlates of individuals who did poorly on our cancellation tests, and found this occurred to a much greater extent in people with visual field defects. Such patients often showed gross asymmetries in space, not only on formal tests but also in natural situations. For example, men would appear with their faces only partially shaven, while women would appear with makeup askew. When we examined incident reports which were filed on an annual basis for insurance purposes, there were more reports of accidents with this group of patients. Patients would skip food appearing on a hospital tray. We even found a patient who was not having breakfast in the hospital because breakfast is usually printed on the left side of hospital menus and he simply did not see the left side. Our findings suggested that there is a syndrome of neglect which can have a profound impact on all ADLs and participation in a rehabilitation program.

Having explored the many clinical manifestations of neglect, we wondered if something could be done to ameliorate them. We noticed that if we supplied cuing, patients could alter the way they scanned and achieve greater success. Among the cues which proved particularly helpful were: (1) *Anchoring:* Providing a strong cue at the beginning of the scan, so the patient had a starting point. This could be accomplished by a red dot at the beginning of a line when a patient was asked to read. With practice, the red dot could be faded or replaced. (2) *Pacing:* Having the patient slow the response, by reciting aloud the target stimuli. This is useful in dealing with impulsivity, the patient's tendency to respond too rapidly, and thereby lose sight of the goal of the task. (3) *Feedback:* Providing appropriate knowledge of results is very useful for an individual who has difficulty knowing whether the answer is correct. (4) *Reducing the information load or task demand:* by having the patient cancel a single, versus a double or triple or conditional target. (5) *Practice:* Rehearsal is important for taking away the novelty of an action by familiarizing the person with all of the elements of a task. Providing people with such cues vastly improved their performance. The results of practice with this approach improved skills in reading and other academic areas involving two dimensional space such as written arithmetic when it is necessary to carry over figures from one column to the next. One of the major virtues of the approach was that it addressed an important clinical point. Patients who omit targets in space tend to be unaware of the presence of a visual perceptual problem. Consequently, it may often be difficult to engage in a problem for which they see no need to remediate. The stimulus materials may therefore have to be quite dramatic and meaningful to engage the patient and convince him that a problem exists. A typical demonstration might be by using money. If large bills are laid out in front of the patient's left half of hemispace, and small coins are placed to the right, and the patient is asked to pick up the money, many may pick up the coins and ignore the larger bills. When the error is pointed out to the patient, he begins to understand that a problem might exist. Furthermore, when he is asked or forced to turn his head to see the money from the right half of his visual field, it is clear that there are solutions to the visual perceptual problem. The patient senses that he is not crazy, and does not have to be embarrassed by failure.

In a series of studies carried out over a decade with positive results, which were replicated by others, we were able to show the benefits of a training program incorporating the techniques and the principles behind the cuing system. We also made the point that when improvement occurred it took place for those activities which were highly similar to the tasks involved in the original training. All the studies included control groups who were matched with experimental groups (Weinberg et al., 1979; 1982). In a followup study to assess the long term effects of the treatment, training benefits were maintained, although the control group was tending to catch up with the experimental group (Gordon et al., 1985). While the training had speeded up recovery, gains could have been even greater if booster shots had been added. Training was aimed at altering premorbid-looking habits. New habits require considerable practice until they become incorporated in the individual's repertoire, in an automatic, effortless way.

However, even more striking observations appeared at followup. Both experimental and control groups appeared socially isolated, seldom venturing out of the house, with time spent on passive recreational activities. They were depressed. Depression in stroke deserves some comment because it may be masked by the individual's difficulty in understanding or expressing emotion, or aprosodia. Perceptual retraining was helpful, but major behavioral and psychological problems persisted. This led to a further series of studies which indicated that perceptual problems typically coexist with depression and underarousal. A perceptual problem seldom existed in isolation. A total treatment package had to broaden the modalities being treated.

We therefore undertook another study, to take into account the multidimensional nature of the problems following stroke. This study featured the following: Graduate students were trained as coaches to deliver perceptual training and to teach caregivers, generally spouses, how to recognize and manage perceptual problems. Students were taught to serve as counselors for family and marital strains, which tend to be aggravated following a stroke. The students worked under the supervision of an experienced psychologist who was familiar with both perceptual retraining and family therapy. The approach to family therapy was "solution-focused" (Simon et al., 1991). In solution-focused therapy there is an assumption that every person has resources which can be utilized. Every patient and every family member has preferences. Each problem has its exceptions. For example, if a couple fights, there are times when they do not fight. To find differences, one can examine the times when fighting occurs and when it does not. Finally, as one begins to explore the situations, new solutions emerge which had not been readily apparent. When a problem occurred, the parties involved were encouraged to think of circumstances with no problems, or of problem circumstances in which solutions had been found. The coaches visited the homes of an "experimental" group of patients, but did not visit the homes or deliver treatment to a control group. The coach might therefore serve as a perceptual remediator, as an escort to take the patient for an outing for a community experience (many patients are afraid to leave their homes) to enhance community integration skills, and as a counselor to assist a caregiver in resolving a problem.

The results indicated that the experimental group appeared to be helped more than the control, in terms of being less depressed and going out of the house more. The methods seemed useful and practical. However, there were a number of caveats about the study which should be mentioned. The results fell short of statistical significance partly because the number of cases who were able to complete the study was small. The groups were not well matched because there were significantly more right brain damaged patients in the experimental group and more left brain damaged cases in the control group (Diller and Simon, 1991).

From our studies, stretching out close to three decades, we draw some conclusions. Individuals can be helped when they have suffered stroke, resulting in damage to the right cerebral hemisphere, and when they present with problems in perception, poor motivation due to underarousal, and/or depression. There are principles which can be applied to relieve caregiver burdens. Our current home service delivery system does not provide ways of dealing with these complex problems. The principles and the techniques offer powerful tools.

BIBLIOGRAPHY

Diller, L., Ben-Yishay, Y., Gerstinan, L.J., Goodkin, R., Gordon, W. & Weinberg, J. (1974). Studies in cognition and rehabilitation in hemiplegia (Rehabilitation Monograph No. 50). New York: New York University Medical Center Institute of Rehabilitation Medicine.

Diller, L. & Simon, D. (1991). Final Report to NIDRR on Grant # 133A8057-88–Psychological and Social Outcome After Stroke.

Diller, L. & Weinberg, J. (1985). Learning from failures in perceptual cognitive retraining in stroke. In B. Uzzell & Y. Gross (eds.), *Clinical neuropsychology of intervention.* Boston: Martinus Nijhoff Publishing.

Gordon, W., Ruckdeschel-Hibbard, M.R., Egelko, S., Diller, L., Shaver, M., Lieberman, A. & Ragnarrson, K. (1985). Perceptual remediation in patients with right brain damage: A comprehensive program. *Archives of Physical Medicine and Rehabilitation, 66,* 353-359.

Simon, D., Kaplan, E., & Diller, L. (1991). Solution-focused intervention with families of cognitively impaired stroke patients. Workshop presentation at the 99th Annual Convention of the American Psychological Association at San Francisco, CA.

Weinberg, J., Diller, L., Gordon, W.A., Gerstruan, L.J., Lieberman, A., Lakin, P., Hodges, G. & Ezrachi, O. (1979). Training sensory awareness and spatial organization in people with right brain damage. *Arch Phys Med Rehab, 60,* 491-496.

Weinberg, J., Piasetsky, E., Diller, L. & Gordon, W. (1982). Treating perceptual organization deficits in non-neglecting RBD stroke patients. *Journal of Clinical Neuropsychology, 4,* 59-75.

Stroke as Chronic Illness:
Living to the Fullest

Fay W. Whitney

Stroke survivors account for 50% of acutely hospitalized neurologic patients (Congressional Budget Office, 1991), 60% of rehabilitation patient populations, and more than 75% of long-term beds (Cry & Duncker, 1992). Yet, 75% of all stroke survivors receive care in the community from family and friends. The number of stroke survivors per year who are permanently disabled or severely impaired in activities of daily living (ADL) totals about 6,969 (Hing & Bloom, 1991). They are at increased risk of institutionalization (West, 1991). The combined costs of medical care and lost wages of stroke survivors are estimated at $4.4 billion per year. We do not know what contribution to cost of care for stroke survivors informal caregivers represent, but it is substantial (Kemper, 1992). Yet, it is striking how little is really known about how stroke survivors and their families live, the problems they face, their quality of life, disappointments and joys (Adkins, 1993; Doolittle, 1988; Whitney, Shaughnessy & Siegler, in press).

There are several reasons for this. First, in the acute phase and immediate rehabilitation, the stroke survivor is institutionalized. This tells us little about how he/she will live at home. Second, home care services and nonacute rehabilitation access is extremely limited (Katov, 1990), unequally distributed (Kemper, 1992) and generally not reimbursed 6-8 weeks following discharge. Third, stable stroke survivor contact with the health care system is infrequent, usually acute or episodic, and highly unorganized. Last, stroke survivors and their families are very good at

Fay W. Whitney, PhD, RN, FAAN, is Associate Visiting Professor at the University of Wyoming, School of Nursing, in Laramie.

[Haworth co-indexing entry note]: "Stroke as Chronic Illness: Living to the Fullest." Whitney, Fay W. Co-published simultaneously in Loss, Grief & Care (The Haworth Press, Inc.) Vol. 8, No. 1/2, 1998, pp. 45-57; and: After Stroke: Enhancing Quality of Life (ed: Wallace Sife) The Haworth Press, Inc., 1998, pp. 45-57. Single or multiple copies of this article are available for a fee from The Haworth Document Delivery Service [1-800-342-9678, 9:00 a.m. - 5:00 p.m. (EST). E-mail address: getinfo@haworth.com].

managing unrelenting difficulties, of "bearing up" and surviving under very burdensome arrangements.

But the fact is, life following stroke survival is not always good. The initial impairments become disabilities over time, and iatrogenic decline is all too common. Poor coordination of services, a maze of inconsistent practices in handling the health needs of elderly disabled adults, and the emphasis on the disease aspects of stroke undermine efforts to help stroke survivors live life to the fullest.

Stroke is viewed as an acute, catastrophic event. Major professional and financial resources are used to help the patient recover fundamental daily function. Yet, many of the basic, daily needs of stroke survivors and families are missed. The literature has conflicting evidence of the long term value of acute rehabilitation intervention designed to regain function (Garraway, Akhtar, Hockey & Prescott, 1980; Indredavik, Bakke, Solberg, Rokseth, Haaheim & Holme, 1991; Stevens, Ambler & Warren, 1984; Wood-Dauphine, Shapiro, Bass, Fletcher, Georges, Heneby and Mendelsohn, 1984). It is nearly silent regarding the value of lifelong recovery and the role of ongoing therapy. Empirically, clinicians see that stroke survivors can continue to improve substantially throughout many years. Conversely, stroke survivors have greater difficulty in maintaining health and preventing the ravages of deconditioning (Clark & Murray, 1988; Siebens, 1990). Present reimbursement policies for long term therapies to prevent deconditioning require evidence of continued improvement, ignoring the equally important need for maintenance and prevention of deconditioning. Much of stroke care is focused on acute intervention, prolonging vital function, and finite rehabilitation strategies. But therapies designed to regain function do not necessarily address major problems encountered by stroke survivors and their families. For instance, there is little intervention available for behavior management, family counseling, respite services, supplemental home care services for the elderly, transportation difficulties, health maintenance and primary or secondary prevention services.

Our care of stroke survivors needs a new focus. Stroke, once survived, produces a chronic illness characterized by: (1) underlying disease with the possibility of chronic exacerbations; (2) the possibility of early or untimely death; (3) long term management requiring integrated control of both present illnesses and prevention of future problems; (4) the effects it has on the way life is lived; and (5) requiring the entire family unit to respond.

The acute disabilities of stroke survivors are generally apparent: losses in motor, sensory, perceptual, language, cognitive and coordination systems are noted. Loss of visual and hearing problems secondary to aging compound the disability and loss of function of stroke survivors (Rudberg, Furner, Dunn & Cassel, 1993). The more chronic problems surface, once the major deficits have improved and function increases. Among the most common problems are physiological deconditioning, depression and loss of motivation, variable levels and quality of family and social support, comorbidities, and loss of social interaction (Adkins, 1993).

Stroke survivors are very vulnerable to deconditioning. The disabilities caused by a stroke (i.e., paralysis, aphasia, dysphagia, ataxia, perceptual and behavioral deficiencies, and depression) when added to a premorbid sedentary life style and comorbidities, can severely limit activity (Siebens, 1990; Rusin, 1990). The result is a sinusoidal course of recovery and exacerbation as the chronic disease progresses. Improvement follows rehabilitation, but deconditioning and loss of functional gains often lead to renewed hospitalization. Once hospitalized, the therapies are re-introduced, and function improves. Following discharge, the decline often begins again, once formal therapies end.

As the individual survives and reorganizes life, premorbid personality, behavior and coping mechanisms again become visible. Family conflict and disorganization are common (Rusin, 1990: Perlin, Mullan, Semple, & Skaff 1990). The reversal of roles, new dependence, fear of possible death, and the need to physically reorient the family system causes formidable stresses within its organizational structure. Psychiatric morbidity, including agitation and depression are often caused by vascular cerebral deficits, and are linked to psychosocial and environmental mediators which can be compounded by family conflict (Cohen, Eisdorfer, Gorelick, Paveza, Luchins, Freels, Ashford, Semla, Levy & Herschman, 1993).

There are more difficulties. Financial problems, interlaced with a new and urgent need to maneuver within a confusing health care system brings on crises and feelings of loss of control. Responsibility for continued life-long therapy is rarely transferred to the stroke survivor from the rehabilitation setting (Whitney, Shaughnessey & Siegler, in press), yet families are expected to respond as though it had been. Old stresses in old relationships can magnify, increasing the concern about abuse, dissolution of marriages, conflict and confrontation. It is not unusual for home care providers to find a family in chaos, instances of child, elder and spouse abuse, neglect—both physical and psychological, poor crisis management, job loss and financial exigencies with inability to organize even small amounts of personal care for either stroke survivor or family members. Instances of caregiver stress are legend in homes where disabled elderly reside, resulting in early nursing home placement.

The enormity of problems encountered in the chronic stages of stroke recovery can seem overwhelming. But, studies have shown that coordination of services in the home after hospital discharge can increase and maintain a patient's functional level, can result in greater patient and family satisfaction, and can require less use of acute care hospitals and nursing homes (Edelstein & Lang, 1991; Jones, Densen & Brown, 1989; Kemper, 1992). In fact, the stroke population is a chronically ill population whose major needs are for nursing care, whose need for medical, rehabilitation therapies and acute care services is intermittent, who basically require coordination of services in an unwieldy system, and who can respond to interventions that maximize the potential of the stroke survivor and family. This set of circumstances led to the development of a model of care the author labels a "rehabilitation team without walls." A description of the model and the outcomes of a pilot research program follow.

THE POST-STROKE CONSULTATION SERVICE

The impetus for the development of this service arose from a funded longitudinal research project (NIH, Institute of Nursing Research) which studied the trajectory and role of depression in stroke. Visits in the homes of stroke survivors revealed the multitude of problems described above. Initiated in 1989, the Post-Stroke Consultation Service provides comprehensive assessment and intervention in the home for stroke survivors and their families. Using a caremanaged format (Association of Rehabilitation Nurses, 1990), a nurse practitioner provided physical, mental, neurological, home safety, rehabilitation and environmental assessment to determine the needs of the stroke survivor and family. In concert with colleagues in geriatrics, physiatry, physical therapy and social work, the nurse practitioner used an interdisciplinary team approach to create a coordinated plan of care in the home that the family could foster and maintain. A prime element in the design was the incorporation of the stroke survivor and family as part of the "rehabilitation team without walls," and ultimately, a transfer of responsibility for the ongoing therapeutic regimen to them. Health screening, primary care health promotion, referral and resource development for the disabled persons and their families were part of the service. The philosophy of case management by the nurse practitioner fused both the economic and individual care management concepts, with an emphasis on efficient and effective use of services and providers, maximizing health outcomes, and putting the stroke survivor and families in control of the endeavor.

Care was delivered in an outpatient clinic, in the hospital, long-term care facility, or at home. The practice used additional services through normal referral networks, and collaborated with existing primary care providers where they existed. Details of the practice can be found elsewhere (Whitney, Shaughnessey & Siegler, in press). Specific services provided included: individual evaluations (history, physical examination, diagnostic testing), periodic monitoring of neurological and physical conditions, medication review and instruction, evaluation and recommendations for exercise programs, identification and referral to community services, home safety assessment, long term care planning, caregiver assessment and crisis counseling. The service was collaborative and cooperative among providers who had interest in geriatrics, stroke rehabilitation, family empowerment, and team building. It has been successful in providing coordinated services for stroke survivors and their families for over nine years, to date.

PILOT RESEARCH

The Post-Stroke Consultation Service became the nidus for a funded pilot research program in 1990. The nurse practitioner in the home found that both active and passive range of motion exercises, transfer techniques, walking and bathroom use decrease markedly, or ceased after discharge from acute care. Deconditioning was not only prevalent, but often was the precursor to stroke survivors becoming either wheelchair dependent or bedridden, even when neurological defects did not correlate with the degree of decreased mobility. The purpose of the pilot grant was to further develop a collaborative practice model, focusing upon the problem of deconditioning due to lack of exercise and the apparent inability to maintain function in the home, following stroke.

SAMPLE

A convenience sample of 15 stroke survivors and their families was recruited from referrals to the Post-Stroke Consultation Service. Those included (1) had evidence of, or risk for deconditioning affecting capacity for ADLs; (2) were medically stable; (3) had no current, formal physical therapy services; and (4) were interested in participation. Excluded were (1) those with cognitive deficits affecting ability to learn exercises; (2) those with perceptual or physical problems that make exercise dangerous; (3) behavior that inhibits consistent cooperation; and/or (4) had no caregiver, or could not independently sustain an exercise program.

DESIGN

The practice design included four professional providers (nurse practitioner, geriatrician, physiatrist, physical therapist) and the stroke survivor/family core. The coordination of services was centered in the existing Post-Stroke Consultation Service with the nurse practitioner acting as coordinator and care manager. Home visits were made by the nurse practitioner and physical therapist. Office visits were made to the geriatrician/physiatrist. Additional services were accessed through normal referral networks, as needed. Central to the process was the development of consolidated assessment and goal setting plans through team meetings and combined office or home visits. Following consent procedures, a minimum of six visits were made. The person(s) involved in the visits and the content of them are represented in Table 1. The variability of the services offered were dependent upon the individual needs and concerns of the family and stroke survivor.

INSTRUMENTS

Physical/Clinical Measurements

A standard history and physical examination format was used to assess the physical and mental status of the stroke survivors. Special attention was given to a thorough neurological assessment with recording of deficits.

Functional Measurements. Only a brief description of the standardized instruments used is given. All instruments are widely used in clinical research and clinical assessment. The reliability and validity have been assessed repeatedly. Summarization of their parametric qualities can be found in both individual research articles, and more briefly in Kane and Kane, 1981.

Barthel's Index is a ten-item index designed to measure functional status and rehabilitation potential in relation to independence or dependence in ADL Is. The range of scores is from 0-100. A score of 0-45 indicates severe disability; 40-60 moderate disability; 61-95 mild disability, and 100, functional independence.

The Functional Independence Measure (FIM) is a widely used rehabilitation measure, requiring training of raters, but has excellent inter-rater reliability. It was used to account for small gains in functional ability across several domains. It can be used as a change score over time.

The Instrumental Activities of Daily Living Scale (IADL) was used to

TABLE 1. Study Visit Schedule and Content

Site of Visit	Provider(s)	Content of Visit
#1 – Home	Nurse Practitioner, Stroke Survivor, Family	1. Assess physical, emotional, neurological, functional and caregiver needs; Safety and home fitness; ADL, IADL's. 2. Set up MD visit 3. Set up PT visit 4. Establish nursing management plan
#2 – Outpatient Clinic	Geriatrician, Physiatrist, Nurse Practitioner, Stroke Survivor and Family	1. Assess medical problems 2. Establish management regimen, prescribe medical interventions 3. Assess rehabilitation needs 4. Establish rehabilitation regimen/prescribe treatment modalities
#3 – Home	Physical Therapist, Nurse Practitioner, Stroke Survivor and Family	1. Perform physical therapy assessment 2. Develop exercise plan and operationalize rehabilitation/physical therapy modality 3 Continue nursing assessment and management 4. Follow up of medical regimen.
TEAM MEETING AT CLINIC	Nurse Practitioner, Physical Therapist, Geriatrician, Physiatrist, Stroke Survivor and Family	1. Review patient and family needs 2. Coordinate goals and plans 3. Deal with communication and practice problems 4. Review and redemonstrate exercise regimen 5. Discover and deal with new problems 6. Determine the need for other referrals 7. Develop and time table to measure progress

TABLE 1 (continued)

Site of Visit	Provider(s)	Content of Visit
#4 – Home	Physical Therapist, Stroke Survivor and Family	1. Implement the exercise program with return demonstrations and problem solving 2. Operationalize physical therapy prescription further and monitor progress
#5 and #6 – Home	Nurse Practitioner, Stroke Survivor and Family	1. Evaluate return demonstrations of exercise program 2. Reteach and reinforce learning as needed 3. Monitor physical, emotional and social conditions of stroke survivor and family 4. Make new referrals as needed 5. Engage in continued coordination of services.

measure degree of independent functioning within the home. It is a 16 item scale used to rate three categories of ability to perform: dependent, assisted and independent. It produces a score in the range of 48 (independent function) to 16 (dependent function). It has been used extensively in clinical settings as a guide to history taking to estimate the ability of elders to function in the home setting.

Outcome Measures

The outcome measures chosen are those which are commonly associated with estimating successful recovery in stroke populations, change in degree of disability, number of additional injuries, changes in skin integrity, number of hospital admissions, and number of provider visits and placement at 6 months post stroke. The sample size limits the generalizability of the outcomes, but does indicate trends that can be expected in using the model of intervention described.

RESULTS

Demographic and Clinical Data

Our population was comparable with most stroke populations in age and type of stroke, but had more women than men, and more right hemisphere damage (RHD) than left, which is unusual statistically (see Table 2). However, our sample was referred to the service because families/ stroke survivors needed interventions. Typically, RHD patients have more behavioral management problems, and may explain why these referrals to us predominated in this small sample. Interestingly, a third of the stroke survivors were living alone, despite their deficits. All were retired. Clinically, these stroke survivors were quite ill, some bedridden, most with more than two ADL requirements.

Changes in Functional Status

The small data set makes the interpretation of the objective data circumstantial (see Table 3). However, each stroke survivor showed some improvement on one of the scales. There is a trend toward improvement in the Barthel's Index early in recovery, and in IADL at six months. The FIM

TABLE 2. Demographic and Clinical Data

Pt. #	AGE	SITE OF LESION	MAJOR FUNCTIONAL PROBLEM
1	75	Left MCA	Aphasia, Right hemiparesis
2	69	Right MCA	Aphasia, Left hemiparesis
3	72	Right thalamic	Slight aphasia, disorientation
4	73	Right MCA	Mild left hemiparesis
5	62	Right Watershed MCA	Left hemiparesis, dysarthria dysphagia
6	42	Left MCA	Right hemiparesis, sublux dysarthria, cognitive impairment/dementia
7	71	Right thalamic hemorrhage with shunt	Dense left hemiparesis

N = 7 (only those with complete data are reported)
Sex = Males – 2; Females – 5
Age – Mean = 64.2, SD 2.3; Range = 42 – 75
Stroke Type – Thromboembolic = 6
Hemorrhagic = 1

TABLE 3. Changes in Functional Scores at 3 Months and 6 Months
(N = 7)

Measure	3 months	6 months
Mean FIM	+ 1.4	+ 1.4
Mean IADL	− 0.2	+ 0.8
Mean Barthel	+ 2.5	no change

showed improvement that peaked at three months and did not change in six months. Once again, intervention shows equivocal results in relation to both the type of improvement and the timing. Pertinent to this probe into the recovery trajectory of stroke survivors are those who did not complete the six month protocol and were not included in the analyses. Two died, one with a recurrent stroke and cardiovascular collapse. Nine could not continue with the exercise regimen because they were too ill, lost family support needed to complete the exercise regimen, or simply could not maintain vigor in the exercise program for a variety of motivational reasons. It appears that those who can be convinced to continue self-therapy, improve. We lack data to tell us why we fail in coordinated efforts to help stroke survivors maintain or increase gain in function.

Outcome Data

The interventions of the "rehabilitation team without walls" is best seen in the trends for outcome data (see Table 4). It bears repeating that these stroke survivors were quite disabled, and to add that most were two to four years post-stroke event. Yet, four out of seven improved in function over six months time on the exercise regimen, no injuries due to falls or other accidental mishaps occurred, and only one had skin breakdown although three were mainly bedridden. Hospital admissions were about 50%. Although this is disappointing, all were returned to home care following the acute illness. Most had appropriately spaced follow-up visits to providers, and one was referred to a new primary care provider, where none had existed before. Most telling was placement at six months. All remained living at home.

Patient/Family Evaluations

Because our philosophy of team care includes the stroke survivor and family as members, it was important for us to survey these participants

TABLE 4. Outcome Variables–Summary
(N = 7)

Changes in Disability	Number of Injuries
None = 3	None Reported = 7
Improved Function = 4	

Changes in Skin Integrity	Number of Hospital Admissions
None = 6	None = 4
Breakdown Lesion = 1	One = 3

Number of Provider Visits	Placement at 6 months
Every Three Months = 5	Home = 7
Referred for Primary Care = 1	Living Alone = 2
Unable to Track = 1	Frequent Supervision = 2
	24-Hour Supervision = 3

regarding their interpretation of the value of the intervention. A nine-item evaluation form was given to both, the stroke survivor and family, who completed it together (see Table 5). The results show that all participants were glad that they had the opportunity to participate, and that all members of the professional team were "helpful" in their respective roles. The majority felt the exercise program was understandable and realistic, and five out of seven said they would continue, now that the protocol was complete. No one felt that no gain had been made during the course of the protocol.

DISCUSSION

Research lends itself to "proving things," usually using statistical methods, and controlling for as many variables as possible. While this is necessary and fruitful, it is also limiting in approaching complex problems like those of stroke survivors and their families. When reality and clinical variation impinges upon methodology, in research we opt for scientific rigor, tending to exclude from our samples those who would skew the data. We adopt interventions that might be methodologically sound, but clinically unreasonable. This small pilot group shows us that there is need for further study, with improved scientific vigor to sort out those interventions that are most likely to provide the best outcomes for the majority of stroke survivors and their families. But, in attempting to do so, it cannot be ignored that this group of patients benefitted from a model of health care

TABLE 5. "Rehabilitation Team Without Walls" Program Evaluation by Patient/Family

(N = 7)

Comments Regarding Program Evaluation	Yes	Somewhat	No
I. Exercise program was understandable	6	1	0
2. Exercise program was realistic	5	2	0
3. We will continue after the study	5	2	0
4. We notice increased function	3	4	0
5. We were included in the planning	2	5	0
6. We are glad we did this	7	0	0
7. PT was helpful	7	0	0
8. NP was helpful	7	0	0
9. MDs were helpful	7	0	0

delivery that has not been widely replicated or appreciated in the past. We should learn from it, refine it, and continue to understand that people working together, coordinating efforts, can provide the best outcomes in complex health care issues. Further, the Post-Stroke Consultation Service philosophy of making the stroke survivor and family members an integral part of the "rehabilitation team without walls" probably gives its function the best chance for long term success.

FUTURE DIRECTIONS

More health services research needs to be mounted to help in the decision making, during the next decade. Although the present surge in interest for reforming the health care system is laudable, the need for it is decades old. No one knows better than the elderly disabled population what formidable barriers to humane and effective care exist. This model needs to be expanded and tested so stroke survivors can live their lives to the fullest as long as they are able. Hopefully, this is a first step, and others will help to make the trail more visible.

REFERENCES

Adkins, E.R. 1993. "Quality of Life After Stroke: Exposing a Gap in Nursing Literature" *Rehabilitation Nursing*, 18(3): 144-147.

Association of Rehabilitation Nurses. 1990. *The Rehabilitation Nurse Case Manager: Role Description*. Skokie, IL: Association of Rehabilitation Nurses (708/966-3433).

Clark, G.S. & Murray, P.K. 1988. "Rehabilitation of the Geriatric Patient." In J. A. Delisa, *Rehabilitation Medicine: Principals and Practice.* Philadelphia: Lippincott.

Cohen, D. et al. 1993. "Psychopathology Associated with Alzheimer's Disease and Related Disorders." *Journal of Gerontology: Medical Sciences,* 48(6):M 255-260.

Dolittle, N. 1988. "Stroke Recovery: Review of the Literature and Suggestions for Future Research." *Journal of Neuroscience Nursing,* 20(3): 169-173.

Edelstein, H. & Lang, A. 1991 "Posthospital Care for Older People: A Collaborative Solution." *Gerontologist,* 31(2): 267-270.

Garraway, W.M. et al. 1980. "Management of Acute Stroke in the Elderly: Preliminary Results of a Controlled Trial." *British Medical Journal,* 281: 827-829.

Hing, E. & Bloom, B. February 1991. "From NCHS: Long-term Care for the Functionally Dependent Elderly." *American Journal of Public Health,* 81: 223-225.

Indredavik, B. et al. 1991. "Benefit of a Stroke Unit: A Randomized Controlled Trial." *Stroke,* 22: 1026-1031.

Jones, E. W., Densen, P.M., Brown, S.D. 1989. "Posthospital Needs of Elderly People at Home: Findings from an Eight-Month Follow-Up Study." *Health Services Research,* 24(6): 644-664.

Kane, R. A. & Kane, R. L. 1981. *Assessing the Elderly.* Lexington, MA: Lexington Books.

Katov, C. 1990. "Access to Geriatric Rehabilitation Services: A Background Paper." *AARP Public Policy Institute,* Washington, D.C. #9002.

Kemper, P. 1992. "The Use of Formal and Informal Home Care by the Disabled Elderly." *Health Services Research,* 27(4), 421-451.

Ory, M. G. & Duncker, A. P. (Eds.). 1992. *In-Home Care for Older People.* Newbury Park: Sage Publications.

Perlin, L. I. et al. 1990. "Caregiving and the Stress Process: An overview of Concepts and Their Measures." *Gerontologist,* 30: 583-594.

Rudberg, M. A. et al. 1993. "The Relationship of Visual and Hearing Impairments to Disability: An Analysis Using the Longitudinal Study of Aging." *Journal of Gerontology: Medical Sciences,* 48(6): M261-265.

Rusin, M.J. 1990. "Stroke Rehabilitation: A Geropsychological Perspective." *Archives of Physical Medicine and Rehabilitation,* 71: 914-922.

Siebens, H. 1990. "Deconditioning." In B. Kemp, K. Brummel-Smith, & J. Ransdell (Eds.). *Geriatric Rehabilitation.* Boston: College-Hill Press.

Stevens, R. S., Ambler, N. R., & Warren, M. D. 1984. "A Randomized Controlled Trial of a Stroke Rehabilitation Ward." *Age and Ageing,* 13: 65-75.

West, J. 1991. "The Americans with Disabilities Act: From Policy to Practice." *The Milbank Quarterly,* 69: Supplement 1/2.

Wood-Dauphinee, W. et al. 1984. "A Randomized Trial of Tea Care Following Stroke." *Stroke,* 15: 864-872

Whitney, F., Shaugnnessey, M., Siegler, E. in press. In E. Siegler & F. Whitney, *Collaborative Practice in Care of the Elderly and Adults.* Springer Publishers.

How Common Is Depression Following Stroke?

Ivan K. Goldberg

On the internet, the particular part of cyberspace that I inhabit fairly regularly, there are a number of documents known as FAQ's. These are answers to Frequently Asked Questions. In this presentation I decided to write an FAQ on the subject of post-stroke depression. A number of studies on the frequency of strokes following depression varied in their estimates, from 22 to 60 percent. The prevalence of depression is greatest between six and twenty-four months post-stroke. In some studies, 25 percent of stroke patients were found to be depressed during the acute stage.

Some stroke patients awaken from a coma in a depressed state. Others develop depression during a period of hospitalization, and others may develop depression months after having had a stroke. In one study of the six-month period following a stroke, the prevalence of major depression increased from 23 to 34 percent, while the frequency of diastema disorder increased from 20 to 26 percent.

Q. What is the relationship between pre-stroke psychiatric factors and the development of poststroke depression?

A. Older age and a family history of anxiety disorder were associated with the development of major post-stroke depression. The severity of the

Ivan K. Goldberg, MD, is Associate in Clinical Psychiatry, College of Physicians and Surgeons, at Columbia University, NY. He is also Executive Director of the New York Pharmacologic Institute.

[Haworth co-indexing entry note]: "How Common Is Depression Following Stroke?" Goldberg, Ivan K. Co-published simultaneously in *Loss, Grief & Care* (The Haworth Press, Inc.) Vol. 8, No. 1/2, 1998, pp. 59-62; and: *After Stroke: Enhancing Quality of Life* (ed: Wallace Sife) The Haworth Press, Inc., 1998, pp. 59-62. Single or multiple copies of this article are available for a fee from The Haworth Document Delivery Service [1-800-342-9678, 9:00 a.m. - 5:00 p.m. (EST). E-mail address: getinfo@haworth.com].

depression was associated with the same factors, as well as with higher pre-stroke neuritis.

Q. What are some of the factors that increase the likelihood of post-stroke depression?

A. Among the factors that increase the likelihood of a post-stroke depression are left anterior brain lesions, dysphasia, and living alone. In another study, post-stroke depressions were associated with reduced cerebral blood flow in the right parieto-occipital regions, and in the anterior temporal and frontal regions of the left hemisphere. It has also been demonstrated that individuals with pre-existing subcortical atrophy and mildly enlarged ventriculars are at an increased risk for the development of post-stroke depression. Some, mostly older studies, have not demonstrated the relationship between left hemisphere strokes and the likelihood of depression.

Q. What is the relationship between the severity of functional impairment and the severity of post-stroke depression?

A. The severity of post-stroke depression is not associated with the severity of stroke induced functional impairment, as measured by activities of daily living, motor strength or severity of aphasia. There is no correlation between the volume of brain tissue destroyed by the stroke and the severity of depression.

Q. How well do non-psychiatric physicians recognize that stroke patients may be depressed?

A. In a study by Schubert et al., 15 stroke patients were evaluated for depression, by psychiatric interview and by a self-report paper and pencil scale. Charts were examined for evidence of detection of depression by the rehabilitation team. Sixty-eight percent were diagnosed as depressed, following psychiatric evaluation. Fifty percent reported significant depression on the Beck Depression Inventory, while none of the patients were described as depressed in any of the chart notes of the rehabilitation team.

Q. What techniques are useful in detecting post-stroke depression?

A. Depression in patients with strokes may be detected by the use of standard psychiatric interviews, semi-structured psychiatric interviews such as the Center for Epidemiological Study Depression Scale and the

Hamilton Depression Scale, and on self-report instruments such as the Beck Depression Scale.

Q. Is there anything that distinguishes post-stroke depressions from the depressions that follow other severe physical illnesses?

A. There have been studies of individuals who developed depressions after strokes, mild cardiac infarctions and spinal cord injuries. Depressed stroke patients were found to have significantly more anxiety than depressed cardiac or spinal cord injury patients.

Q. Is there any way to predict which stroke patients will still be depressed in three years?

A. Stroke patients who were found to have hyperadrenocorticism, as manifested by nonsuppression and Dextermethozone Suppression Tests administered three months after their strokes demonstrated a high probability of being depressed three years later. This predictive tool has a sensitivity of 70 percent and specificity of 97 percent.

Q. How does depression affect the cognitive functioning of stroke patients?

A. Major depression in stroke patients is associated with cognitive changes that may make the patient appear to be suffering from severe dementia. When such patients recover from their depressions, their appearance may greatly improve. Among patients with left hemisphere lesions, those with major depression perform significantly below non-depressed patients, on tests of cognitive ability. In patients with right hemisphere lesions, those with depression did not perform below nondepressed patients on tests of cognitive functions.

Q. What is the relationship between post-stroke depression and a successful rehabilitation?

A. The depressed stroke patients progress less well in rehabilitation than non-depressed stroke patients. Because of this, it is of great importance that depression screening be a part of the management of people who have suffered strokes. Depression was associated with only one-half the improvement in functional stasis found in non-depressed patients with failure to improve cognitive performance and with deterioration in physical capacity over time. Patients with post-stroke depression were found to be less likely to resume social activities than patients without such depressions.

Q. What is the relationship between depression and death in stroke patients?

A. In a study of 84 stroke patients, only 2 percent of the non-depressed patients died. Ten percent of the patients with minor depressions died, and 23 percent of the patients with major depression died. Depression is not highly correlated with severity of the stroke. It appears that depression is an independent risk factor for death, in stroke survivors.

Q. Is post-stroke mania associated with any particular lesion?

A. Post-stroke mania is associated with dysfunction of the basal temporal cortex in the right hemisphere.

Q. Is the easy laughing and crying that is seen in some individuals with a stroke caused by their being depressed or manic?

A. While some patients with inappropriate laughing or crying may be depressed or in an elated mood, most are not. The disregulation of laughing or crying can occur without any symptoms of a mood disorder. The Pathological Laughter and Crying Scale is a reliable and valid method for measuring such behavior.

Q. Have anti-depressants been found to be a useful treatment for patients with post-stroke depressions?

A. Tricyclic anti-depressants, especially Nortriptyline, selected serotonin reup-taker inhibitors, especially Fluoxetine and the reversible monoamine oxidase, Moclobemial, have been used successfully to treat such patients. Their useful-ness has been established in double-blinded placebo controlled clinical trials. For psycho-stimulants such as Methylphenidate, Ritalin is useful as a treatment for depressed stroke patients. In order to avoid some of the side effects associated with treatment using conventional anti-depressants, a group of ten depressed stroke patients were treated by Johnson et al. with Methylphenidate in an open label design. Improvement was noticed in seven patients. This result needs to be replicated in a placebo-controlled double-blinded study.

Q. What psycho-social factors seem to be important in recovery from post-stroke depression?

A. One factor that has been identified to be of great importance in facilitating the recovery from post-stroke depression is the patient's perception of adequate social support. Patients who perceive social support to be inadequate, particular-ly from a spouse caregiver, are at risk of a longer duration of depression.

Q. What treatments are effective in a patient who exhibits pathological laughing, following a stroke?

A. Pathological laughing and crying after a stroke usually respond to treat-ment with antidepressants. Tricyclic antidepressants and selected Crytones reuptake inhibitors have been shown to be effective.

Stroke and Quality of Life:
Intimacy and Sexuality Poststroke

Linda Chadwick
Jeffrey Saver
Jose Biller
Jenifer Carr

Members of the Stroke Program at the Northwestern University Medical School investigated the resumption of poststroke sexual activity/intimacy and its importance to stroke patients and their sexual partners. A basic data demographic form, individual patient and partner questionnaires, and the Beck Depression Inventory were mailed to 46 participants involved in past or present clinical trials. Twenty-seven patients responded (16 men, 10 women, 1 gender unknown) along with nineteen partners (8 men, 11 women).

Dependent variables included current sexual activity, length of time between stroke onset and sexual activity resumption, and level of importance. Ten patients had not resumed sexual activity. Seventeen patients had reestablished a sexual relationship. Both patients and partners, stated poststroke sexual education was not received. This lack of sexual education warrants further investigation.

Linda Chadwick, BSN, RN, is Coordinator of the Stroke Program, as well as Administrative Officer for Research, Department of Neurology at Indiana University Medical Center. Jose Biller, MD, is Professor and Chairman, Department of Neurology, Indiana University Medical Center. Jeffrey Saver, MD, is Director of Stroke Services at UCLA Department of Neurology, at Los Angeles and Jenifer Carr is Coordinator of Alternative Programs at Northwestern Medical Faculty Foundation in Chicago.

[Haworth co-indexing entry note]: "Stroke and Quality of Life: Intimacy and Sexuality Poststroke." Chadwick, Linda et al. Co-published simultaneously in *Loss, Grief & Care* (The Haworth Press, Inc.) Vol. 8, No. 1/2, 1998, pp. 63-69; and: *After Stroke: Enhancing Quality of Life* (ed: Wallace Sife) The Haworth Press, Inc., 1998, pp. 63-69. Single or multiple copies of this article are available for a fee from The Haworth Document Delivery Service [1-800-342-9678, 9:00 a.m. - 5:00 p.m. (EST). E-mail address: getinfo@haworth.com].

Of all the parameters that determine quality of life after stroke, sexuality is the most neglected. The sexual lives of stroke patients and partners are frequently overlooked in formal scientific studies of life satisfaction after stroke, and in bedside counseling of stroke patients by physicians, nurses, physical and occupational therapists, and other caregivers. Sexuality is a vital facet of normal living, not only for young stroke victims but also for older individuals who are disproportionately afflicted by cerebrovascular insults. The World Health Organization has defined sexual health as "the integration of the somatic, emotional, mental and social aspects of sexual being, in ways that are positively enriching and that enhance personality, communication, and love" (Calderone 1981:131). Any analysis of quality of life after stroke is fundamentally unsound if it fails to encompass the sexual life of stroke patients. This pilot study is aimed to identify and examine intimacy and sexuality among stroke patients and their partners.

METHODS

For this study a basic data demographic form, a questionnaire for both the stroke patient and partner, and the Beck Depression Inventory for the stroke patient were mailed (two separate mailings) to 46 participants involved in past or present stroke clinical trials.

Participants had had an ischemic stroke within the past three years and all were living at home. Nineteen patients and 14 partners responded to the first mailing. After a second mailing, eight additional patients and five additional partners responded.

Dependent variables included outcome measures established to reflect the stroke patients' quality of life, in regard to the importance of intimacy and poststroke sexuality. Variables were determined by (1) current sexual activity, (2) length of time between onset of stroke and resumption of sexual activity, and (3) importance of sexual activity/intimacy. Independent variables were obtained from the Beck Depression Inventory, and were used as an indicator to detect unknown coping difficulties.

RESULTS

Twenty-seven patients with stroke replied (16 men, 10 women, one did not return the basic data demographic form, and the gender is unknown). Ages ranged from 36 to 75 for men (mean age range = 66-75), and 36 to

75 for women (mean age range = 56-65) (Table 1). Eighteen patients were married, two widowed, one divorced, and five were single. Two of the single patients had sexual partners outside the home. Associated risk factors are listed in Table 2. Nineteen partners (8 men, 11 women) also completed the form, although one partner answered only three of the questions.

All patients had mild to moderate residual effect from the stroke. All were independent to partially dependent, with five receiving outpatient physical therapy. The interval between stroke onset and their response was between three and thirty-six months.

Changes in sleep pattern as well as increased irritability were the changes most noted by patients, according to the Beck Depression Inventory. Fifteen reported no change in sexual interest, six had a slight decrease in interest, four noted a major decrease in interest, and two noted a total lack of interest in sex.

Seventeen patients had resumed a sexual relationship, ten had not, and one of the patients indicated that the partner was responsible for the lack of sexual relationship. Of those who were currently sexually active, most had resumed the relationship less than three months, poststroke. Eleven patients had reestablished other forms of intimacy (kissing, touching, etc.) while six had not. Nine felt the level of intimacy was not the same as it was prior to stroke. Six patients expressed dissatisfaction with either the intimate or sexual aspects of their relationships.

Patients and partners were asked to rank the importance of sexual intimacy to them. Twelve ranked it as not important, four as important, and eleven as very important. Only two patients expressed concern that a sexual relationship might aggravate their stroke or be the precipitant of a recurrent stroke. Nine patients expressed concern about how their stroke may affect their sexual function, yet only two ranked their stress level as severe after resuming sexual activities. Although 14 patients indicated that their sleep pattern had changed, only six felt they were emotionally fatigued. These factors appear to be related to a change in self-image as 15 patients responded that the stroke had affected the way they thought about themselves. Four had feelings of social isolation.

All subjects stated they did not receive any poststroke sexual education from physicians, nurses, or therapists at the hospital, rehabilitation center, or outpatient clinic. The questionnaire given to the partners had additional questions regarding their role as caretakers. Partners were asked whether they believed stroke itself was the greatest obstacle to reestablishing sexual contact. Seven partners indicated that sexuality was not important to them, eight felt it was important, and four indicated it was very important.

TABLE 1. Mean Age Range

AGE RANGE	MEN	WOMEN
18-25	0	0
26-35	0	0
36-45	1	1
46-55	4	2
56-65	3	4
66-75	6	3
75 or Older	2	0
Mean Age Range	66-75	56-65

TABLE 2. Risk Factors

RISK FACTOR	MEN	WOMEN
HYPERTENSION	8(50%)	8(80%)
DIABETES	5(31.2%)	5(50%)
HEART DISEASE	6(37.5%)	0
HYPERLIPIDEMIA	5(31.2%)	2(20%)
OTHER	1(6.2%)	4(40%)

Partners denied emotional fatigue, changes in sleep pattern, feelings of social isolation, and were not afraid that sexual activity could make their companion's condition worse, or cause another stroke. While none of the partners received education regarding poststroke sexual contact, several indicated that counseling in this area would be helpful.

DISCUSSION

A stroke is an all-encompassing illness. Anxieties run rampant for the stroke patient, family members, and friends. These anxieties are often heightened by a lack of knowledge about the disease process and what to expect during recovery (Rosenthal 1993). The health care team is often very attentive, and seems to concentrate its efforts mainly during the acute stroke phase. Most of the follow-up care is conducted by therapists, yet too often none of these professionals discuss relevant issues, regarding poststroke sexuality.

In the 1970s, in particular, there was a major lack of sexual information for the stroke patient. A decade later, more information became available and open communication about sexuality poststroke was beginning to occur (Daniels 1981). In the 1990s, more attention is being given to this important topic. Very scanty literature is available and very few members of the health care team discuss sexuality with the stroke patient and the sexual partner. Similarly, articles discussing poststroke quality of life issues seem to concentrate primarily on the reestablishment of work and social activities. Very few emphasize reestablishment of an intimate sexual relationship. And even fewer discuss the effect of stroke on the sexual partner.

However, some investigators have examined the sexual life of stroke patients. Bray investigated the sexual interest, function, and attitudes of 35 patients before and after stroke (Bray 1981). He demonstrated no significant change in sexual interest or desire. Our study arrived at similar conclusions.

Monga evaluated 113 stroke patients; personal interviews were conducted with 75 patients and their spouses (Monga 1986). Both men and women had a decline in libido, poststroke. The most common factor cited as responsible for decline in sexual activity was fear that sexual activity might adversely affect blood pressure and cause another stroke. Other aspects of sexual behavior, such as touching, were not examined. Unlike Monga's study, our study found only a slight decrease in intimacy, after stroke.

As Renshaw observed, "Stroke is indeed an emotional word, conjuring up visual images of wheelchairs, walkers, catheters, canes, splints, speech problems, and drooling facial paralysis" (Renshaw 1975: 68). This image of permanent disability does not generally acknowledge the possibility of returning to work and social activities, much less of reestablishing sexual activity.

Each component of sexuality (sexual function, self-image, and interpersonal relations) needs to be carefully evaluated (Bronstein 1991). The questionnaire developed for our study addressed these areas of concern. The stroke itself may alter any or all of these factors. There may be a new self-image, a change in libido, or difficulty with interpersonal relationships; the stroke may have caused aphasia, hemiparesis or sphincteric disturbances.

Bonding together after a stroke may be difficult for the patient and the partner and they often become preoccupied with rehabilitation, in order to regain as much independent function as possible. How often they inquire about reestablishing a sexual relationship, and how often they are offered information is unknown.

Emphasis on psychosocial reentry needs to be as high a priority as physical rehabilitation. Since ischemic stroke primarily affects the population older than age 60, concurrent life changes, such as leisure activities, may also be taking place. A stroke involves a major adjustment and extreme individual suffering. However, the stroke survivor should not, because of age, be expected to be unconcerned with the reestablishment of intimacy or a sexual relationship. Some life changes and innovative coping techniques may be required in order to resume a healthy sexual relationship.

Our pilot study shows that there continues to be a well-developed social network after stroke, and this includes sexuality. The partner of the stroke survivor needs to be included in these coping stages. Although some patients and their partners may feel that sexuality is "private business," many indicate a desire for more open communication and education about sexuality, poststroke. Because discussions of sexuality may be embarrassing or uncomfortable, health care professionals need further education and training in approaching the topic of sexuality with their patients.

Our study did not address lesion localization, as we were blinded to the respondents. Other limitations of our study include the small sample size, lack of investigating risk factors and medications, male potency or female decrease in vaginal lubrication, or prestroke issues. The use of the Beck Depression Inventory does not demonstrate if the stroke itself caused the changes.

A follow-up study plans to investigate what type of activities and frequency were engaged in prestroke versus poststroke. In order to quantify the results, a scale ranking the activity may be used.

CONCLUSIONS

Sexuality and intimacy appear more important to stroke survivors than they are to the stroke partner. Sexuality can be dramatically affected following stroke. The stroke survivor may lose self-confidence, be uncertain how to ask for assistance, or may simply give up on a sexual relationship. The sexual partner may also experience these difficulties. As health care professionals, we need to include the subject of sexuality as an integral part of the rehabilitative process.

REFERENCES

Bray, G., De Frank, R.S., Wolfe, T.L. "Sexual Functioning in Stroke Survivors." *Archives of Physical Medicine and Rehabilitation*, 1981; 62: 286-288.

Bronstein, K., Popovich, J., Stewart-Amidei, C. "Alterations in Sexuality." *Promoting Stroke Recovery*. New York: Mosby 1991, pp. 217-238.

Calderone, M. "Sexuality and Disability in the United States." *Sexuality and Physical Disability-Personal Perspectives*. St. Louis: Mosby 1981, 129-132.

Daniels, S. "Critical Issues in Sexuality and Disability." *Sexuality and Physical Disability-Personal Perspectives*, St. Louis: Mosby 1981, 5-10.

Monga, T., Lawson, J., Inglis J., "Sexual Dysfunction in Stroke Patients." *Archives of Physical Medicine and Rehabilitation*, 1986; 67: 19-22.

Renshaw, D. "Sexual Problems in Stroke Patients." *Medical Aspects of Human Sexuality*, 1975; 9(12): 68-74.

Rosenthal, S., Pituch, M., Greninger, L., Metress, E. "Perceived Needs of Wives of Stroke Patients." *Rehabilitation Nursing*, 1993; 18(3): 148-153.

SUGGESTED READING

Allison, M. "The Effect of Brain Injury on Marriage." *Headlines*. May/June 1993: 3-8.

Binder, L. "Emotional Problems After Stroke." *Current Concepts of Cerebrovascular Disease-Stroke*, July-Aug 1983: 174-177.

De Jong, G., Branch, L. G. "Predicting the Stroke Patient's Ability to Live Independently." *Stroke*, 1982; 13(5): 648-655.

Emick-Herring, B. "Sexual Changes in Patients and Partners Following Stroke." *Rehabilitation Nursing*, Mar-Apr 1985: 28-30.

Freda, M., Rubinsky, H. "Sexual Function in the Stroke Survivor." *Physical Medicine and Rehabilitation Clinics of North America*, 1991; 2(3): 643-659.

Goddess, E., Wagner, N. N., Silverman, D.R. "Poststroke Sexual Activity of CVA Patients." *Medical Aspects of Human Sexuality*, March 1979: 22-30.

Montague, A. *Touching, the Human Significance of the Skin*. New York: Harper and Row, 1974.

Renshaw, D. "Intimacy and Intercourse." *Medical Aspects of Human Sexuality*, 1984; 18(2): 70-76.

Renshaw, D. "Sex and the Senior Citizen." *NAPPH Journal*, Sept. 1978: 56-61.

Robinson-Smith, G. "Coping and Life Satisfaction After Stroke." *Journal of Stroke and Cerebrovascular Disease*, 1993; 3(4): 209-215.

Sjogren, K. "Leisure After Stroke." *Int Rehab Med*. 1982;4:80-87.

Sjogren, K. and Fugl-Meyer, A. R. "Adjustment to Life After Stroke with Special Reference to Sexual Intercourse and Leisure." *Journal of Psychosomatic Research*, 1982; 26(4): 409-417.

White, E. "Appraising the Need for Altered Sexuality Information." *Rehabilitation Nursing*, 1986; 11(3): 6-9.

PART II
PROFESSIONAL CONTRIBUTIONS

Nursing Care of the Stroke Patient:
The Essence of Healing

Kathleen M. Dirschel

The key to successful rehabilitation in the patient with stroke is the healing relationship which is initially established between nurse and patient. With this, initiated by both sides, a commitment to healing emerges and the resources of energy and skill, contributed by both, achieve maximum healing for the patient and ultimate excellence in nursing practice.

The role of nursing as a member of the stroke care team is best described as the dynamic force which brings energy for healing, and skill for integrating the multiple clinical services which are necessary for care. Nursing is the glue that holds all the therapies together. The opportunity that the nurse has in the care of the stroke patient is the fullest use of the therapeutic self, in order to maximize physical rehabilitation. This is done

Kathleen M. Dirschel, RN, PhD, is Director of Education at Valley Hospital in Ridgewood, NJ. Prior to this, Dr. Dirschel was Executive Vice President and Chief Nursing Officer at Columbia Presbyterian Medical Center. She holds a post-doctoral certificate from Harvard University, and has served as Dean of Nursing at Seton Hall University, and as president of the New Jersey State Board of Nursing.

[Haworth co-indexing entry note]: "Nursing Care of the Stroke Patient: The Essence of Healing." Dirschel, Kathleen M. Co-published simultaneously in *Loss, Grief & Care* (The Haworth Press, Inc.) Vol. 8, No. 1/2, 1998, pp. 71-78; and: *After Stroke: Enhancing Quality of Life* (ed: Wallace Sife) The Haworth Press, Inc., 1998, pp. 71-78. Single or multiple copies of this article are available for a fee from The Haworth Document Delivery Service [1-800-342-9678, 9:00 a.m. - 5:00 p.m. (EST). E-mail address: getinfo@haworth.com].

71

through the nursing process that includes assessment, planning and coordinating care, clinical action, and evaluating outcomes. However, the therapeutic use of self also includes the imparting of encouragement, understanding, enthusiasm and comfort, so the spirit of the patient is unified and healed even though the therapies are diverse and separated.

There are many modalities which the nurse may use in the creation and process of the healing relationship. This chapter will focus on selected ones which encompass both the clinical care and the therapeutic use of self. In both major areas, knowledge, skill, and commitment on the part of the nurse are paramount. If the modalities are to be effective, however, an intense communication between the spirits of both the patient and the nurse must be established. In essence, in the healing relationship, nurse and patient are soul mates, as recovery progresses.

HISTORICAL PERSPECTIVE

Nursing texts of "old" (20 years or so) dealt with mechanistic, physical rehabilitative approaches, to care. Comments from one such text are reflective of this:

> The rehabilitation of the hemiplegic man or woman may be a long, drawn out process and may be discouraging at times, but it is well worthwhile because with modern rehabilitation a patient with hemiplegia is no longer relegated to bed or to a wheelchair. He may be taught to feed himself, dress himself, get out of bed and walk with assistance of a short leg brace and the use of a cane. . . . The morale of the patient may be given a big boost if he is able to assume responsibility for some of the activities of daily living while still in the hospital . . .[1]

While these comments are not inaccurate, as far as they go, much new knowledge in the areas of clinical skill and therapeutic use of self in creating the healing relationship have significantly elevated and energized the nursing role and the patient's potential for achieving a higher quality of life.

The newer nursing literature focuses on assessment skills of involved clinical systems, the use of a more standardized language to describe symptoms and pathology, and the development of "critical pathways," to guide practice and care through a time based hospital stay, so all modalities of care are given during preselected time frames. In this situation, which is becoming more and more common, the nurse is the "manager" of care, as well as the giver of certain clinical care components. These newer concepts notwithstanding, the nursing literature in the care of the stroke patient is still quite physical-rehabilitation oriented.

The principals and practice of rehabilitation nursing have been more recently described in the following way:

> The most common complications that threaten a patient with a prolonged illness, such as stroke, are contractures, pressure sores, and bladder and bladder problems. The major goals of the nurse in rehabilitation are as follows:
>
> 1. To prevent deformities and complications.
> 2. To motivate, teach and support the patient and his family during the daily activities of living.
> 3. To refer the patient for proper follow-up care and supervision. . . .[2]

As is evident, we are beginning to see the emergence of other thought, which could clearly enhance the concept of nursing care–and thereby the opportunity for improved healing.

THE PHASES OF NURSING CARE

The Acute Phase

As the third leading cause of death in the United States, stroke is a formidable health care problem, costing more than $14 billion annually for related care, by 1990. The multiple and potentially widespread disabilities related to the cerebral-vascular event pose a demanding challenge to nurses and other members of the health care team, to assure that the patient is efficiently stabilized and secondary problems do not arise, or are kept to a minimum. In addition to the physiological management of a profoundly critical event, external factors demanding high technology usage in a cost-conscious environment, which must occur in every shortening length of stay, complicate this already challenging medical emergency.

While it is not the purpose of this paper to provide great detail on the clinical skills needed by nurses at this initial stage of treatment (this material is available in multiple textbooks on the subject) the author would like to briefly summarize the kinds of nursing activities which go on in this phase of monitoring and stabilization, as precedent to healing. Essentially, the nursing role is of frequent, in-depth, neurological assessment which is recorded, trended, reported, and acted on by virtue of protocols, procedures, and direct physician orders. The assessment includes such components as measuring the level of consciousness, pupillary responses, motor and sensory functions, and of course, overall vital signs. These assessments require a high level of skill, understanding of complex technology, and vigilance.

While the assessments are ongoing, the other contemporaneous roles of nursing include the maintenance of complete bed rest (not always easy to do, especially with other clinical services also providing care) and the maintenance of adequate ventilation, which is a major consideration. This would include roles in proper positioning, suctioning, maintenance of artificial airways, and care of patients on ventilatory devices.

At this phase, nursing care is also directed to maintaining perfusion pressures to prevent further hypoxia and ischemia, monitoring and correcting fluid and electrolyte disturbances, a very proactive interdisciplinary effort to avoid nutritional depletion which can significantly affect muscle wasting and skin breakdown, and eventually hospitalization and recovery potential. At this acute stage, nursing care, in coordination with other clinical services, is also focused on maintaining passive mobility, preventing deep vein thromboses, managing bowel and bladder disturbances, and assessing cognitive and communication disorders.

RELATIONSHIP OF CLINICAL MANDATES
AND THE ESSENCE OF HEALING

Even at this critical stage of stroke care, where the case could be made for intensive physiological management to be the full focus of the nursing care, the necessity for the art of nursing through therapeutic use of self emerges as a vital aspect of the caring process. It is so vital, in fact, that without this energy force, the effects of the therapies may be less effective on individual patient needs, and less targeted to patient drive and commitment to achieve.

The competencies for nursing practice in this realm are considerably different from those mentioned earlier. These are relatively new nursing modalities, using more empathic understanding and energy to facilitate the healing process. Some of these competencies have been articulated in works by Benner, Bishop and Scudder, and other authors, as well.

Initiated then, even at the earliest stages, caring competencies are the glue and the catalyst for maximal recovery, which is cared for by a widely diverse health care delivery team. Some of the competencies identified by Benner[3] which are essential to develop are:

1. Creating a Climate for Establishing a Commitment to Healing

This commitment to healing means the relationship is established between nurse and patient, and both are involved and responsible. What is involved here? Primarily, hope must be mobilized for the nurse, as well as for the patient. This is achieved through exploratory commentary with the patient (when able, or one way communication, when possible), or simply by developing a dedicated mindset to finding understanding of the illness, pain or fear. If the nurse develops this mindset alone because of the acuity of the patient, then that is her role, as well as the sharing of that mindset with the patient—perhaps even wordlessly, through therapeutic touch. Assisting in this process would be social, emotional or spiritual support provided by family or professionals, and managed by the nurse so the amount of input is therapeutic and utilized most effectively by the patient.

In this modality the nurse can offer hope and concrete strategies, and utilize her interpretive skills to enable the patient to create a commitment to his/her own healing.

A second competency which the nurse could develop which is especially useful in the acute phase of stroke care is:

2. Providing Comfort Measures and Preserving Personhood in the Face of Pain and Extreme Breakdown

In the situation where the patient is so ill that little can be done to prolong life, there is often some room to enhance the quality of life, however short it may be. Of particular focus in situations like this is that the nurse must not avoid the humanness of the patient, and must still find ways of providing comfort for him and his family.[3] Here is a quote from a nurse using this competency:

> . . . She was my patient. And you know just because she was so severely ill from the stroke that they cannot do anything else for her doesn't mean that I stop caring for her. So I gave her a bath. She had her little suitcase with her so I put her in one of her gowns and propped her up all around in her bed with pillows. I didn't feel that I was doing anything special for her. But the son told me at the end how much it meant to him . . .[4]

With this nursing practice the mindset of "doing for" and "curing" contributes to and facilitates the patient's sense of personhood, meaning and dignity.

There are many other competencies which form the glue and the energy of healing, and some more will be discussed here. It is important to set the stage to observe the patient as he/she moves into a more stabilized physiological state, where the focus of care allows for more active rehabilitation. The health care team will still be multi-disciplinary, although other disciplines may now enter the therapeutic arena. And the roles of some team members may change, as well. The nurse is an example of one of the team members whose role will modify in the rehabilitation focus phase. The therapeutic approach at this phase is the utilization of active rehabilitation nursing principles and practice. The physical functions which rehabilitation nursing focuses on are balance, posture, muscle tone, movement sensation and perception. These functions are also the core of the specialized therapies, such as physical therapy and occupational therapy. Nursing has the special role of coordinating these practices, reinforcing, and interdependently practicing them.

While implementing selected exercises and movements based on these functions, it is key to remember that positioning and guided practice techniques help the patient relearn postural balancing, and function more safely. Since unconscious postural reactions are impaired in the stroke patient, fear of falling is a common problem. Overcoming this by practicing posture and bringing the balance to a cognitive level is therefore a key goal and one in which all the appropriate therapeutic modalities can work together.

It is important to remember that posture, itself, is also impaired. Patients generally turn their head away from the affected side, with their neck tilted toward it. Therapeutic rehabilitation from any clinical group focuses on recreating normal posture by attending to both sides through such activities as rolling over, sitting up and standing up. Balance is a major aspect of posture, so special attention must be paid to relearning this. We focus on two aspects: static balance, which allows a person to maintain an upright posture, and dynamic balance which keeps the person from falling, when performing movement in activities of daily living. In the stroke patient, there are key physiological barriers to achieving balance which must be assessed and managed so that they are reduced. In the stroke patient, muscle tone is abnormal and inhibited, primarily because there are varying degrees of spasticity and flaccidity occurring simultaneously. In addition, excessive effort, fear, pain or abnormal movement may increase spasticity.

The goal of rehabilitative nursing in coordination with other modalities is to achieve a normal level of tone by having the patient maintain a symmetrical posture, and bear weight on the affected side. Skilled guiding techniques are excellent methods used to assist patients to achieve a normal tone, while performing functional activities. Skilled guiding is the placement of the nurse's hand over the patient's affected hand as an assistance with holding objects (combs, for example). Then guidance is given, as the nurse helps the patient through the normal movement pattern needed to accomplish the task. Patients receive sensory feedback and begin building a movement pattern with normal sequence, rhythm and speed. Using this approach keeps patients active, and allows them to experience success in the completion of a meaningful activity. It also encourages the patient to incorporate the affected side in all activities and provides sensory stimulation on the affected side. In this way, bilateral movement (which is normal movement) is facilitated by the rehabilitation nursing process. Through the recovery phase, the nurse will enhance progress by asking the patient to perform more complex functions, while giving verbal, visual and manual guidance.

The performance of the rehabilitation process is demanding, tiring and energy-draining for both nurse and patient. It is important, then, to include in the therapeutic regimen further energy enhancing competencies. These should occur at the same time as the therapies, in a more intensive fashion, and perhaps less intensively at other times, during the caregiving process.

The third competency for nursing practice, according to Benner, is:

3. Presencing: Being with a Patient[5]

Essentially this brings the nurse beyond *doing for* a patient, as is seen in parts of the rehabilitation process, to the state of *being with* a patient. This competency has been described by nurses as a person-to-person thing. It is a feeling of closeness, of real communication—often without verbal communication. It is the commitment to be there, just to listen to somebody expressing his/her concerns. It doesn't necessarily mean having an answer or suggesting a solution.

Being with the patient, the "presence factor" simply means providing comfort for the patient by touch, tenderness, and sharing feelings of self-esteem and self-confidence. The importance of touch in providing comfort can not be overly stressed, and it may be the only avenue of comfort and communication, which is available. Consider this example of the nurse, using touch:

> Elizabeth (the nurse) put a lot of cream on her hands and warned the patient that it was going to be cold, apologizing for it. For a while she used both hands while massaging him. At other times she used her right hand, rubbing him firmly, but obviously, gently. There was not much

conversation at this time . . . The nurse said she liked to use the backrub as a chance to talk to him, in a different way of communication.[6]

By utilizing the above three competencies and the therapeutic use of self, the nurse can better reach the essence of healing, in the rehabilitation process.

The role of the nurse as a vital member of the stroke team is ever changing and improving, as new knowledge is being gleaned. This is an especially exciting era, in which we are witnessing the emergence of new approaches, which are markedly enhancing the concept and quality of nursing care–and the resultant improved healing that must follow. With the high level of skill, vigilance and dedication of nursing, the added personal touch does make a difference.

REFERENCES

1. Terry, Benz et al. *Principals and Techniques of Rehabilitation Nursing*. The C. V. Mosby Co., St. Louis, 1961. p 181.

2. Brunner, L., Suddarth, D. *Textbook of Medical Surgical Nursing*. J. P. Lippincott Co., Philadelphia, PA, 1988. p 217.

3. Benner, P. *From Novice to Expert*. Addison-Wesley Publishing Co., Menlo Park, CA, 1984. pp. 49-75.

4. Op Cit, p. 55.

5. Op Cit, p. 56.

6. Op Cit, p. 63.

Rehabilitation Nursing on a Stroke Unit

Sally Hochrein

The goal for a rehabilitation nurse is to help her stroke patients return to the community, functioning at the best possible level. One of the most important qualities of the nurse is patience. It is much harder to teach patients to tie their shoelaces than it is to just do it for them. Sometimes this can be perceived as not taking care of the immediate needs of the patient. For the moment, tying them would be the quickest and easiest thing to do. But in the long run, it is unproductive. Rehabilitation nurses must follow a "hands off" policy, which is the complete opposite of those working in acute care.

At the Burke Rehabilitation Hospital we have a 30 bed stroke unit. Patients come to us from all walks of life–Sheiks from Saudi Arabia, Nobel Prize winners, people with little education, and even homeless persons. When they first arrive we try to set limited goals for them to accomplish, to minimize their initial frustration.

Nurses assess each stroke patient and set up plans to meet the needs of the individual. Each morning the head nurse gives the doctor a complete listing of the patient's problems. This can include medication requirements, bowel and bladder difficulties, intake and output, rashes, leg edemas, and much more.

In rehabilitation, patient education is our prime focus, and it begins the day of admission. This includes the families, as well as any significant others. In the older population, particularly, the spouses may need a lot of training. We encourage them to come in often, participate in programs, and help us in ADL care.

Sally Hochrein, RN, is a member of the Department of Social Work, Stroke Unit at Burke Rehabilitation Hospital in White Plains, New York.

[Haworth co-indexing entry note]: "Rehabilitation Nursing on a Stroke Unit." Hochrein, Sally. Co-published simultaneously in *Loss, Grief & Care* (The Haworth Press, Inc.) Vol. 8, No. 1/2, 1998, pp. 79-82; and: *After Stroke: Enhancing Quality of Life* (ed: Wallace Sife) The Haworth Press, Inc., 1998, pp. 79-82. Single or multiple copies of this article are available for a fee from The Haworth Document Delivery Service [1-800-342-9678, 9:00 a.m. - 5:00 p.m. (EST). E-mail address: getinfo@haworth.com].

The unit is designed so all therapists, the social worker and the doctor have their offices together. This facilitates greater interaction and teamwork between the disciplines. There are some single rooms to encourage family members to stay over. There are also soundproof, visually monitored rooms for patients who have safety awareness problems. We also have a kitchen, so the patients can be assessed and trained in their meal preparation abilities. At lunch and dinner the patients are brought to our dining room, and monitored for swallowing problems.

Assessment is ongoing, throughout the patient's stay. On the day of admission we take base vital signs, including leg measurements, and weight. And we check for perceptual problems such as neglect, denial, spatial and picture ground deficits. We look for receptive, expressive, global problems, apraxia, cognitive functioning, and do bowel and bladder control assessments, as well as for hearing and vision. Safety awareness is high on our list, and necessary steps may have to be taken to assure a safe environment, such as side rails, wheelchair belts, bumpers and anti-tip devices. For swallowing problems we have three levels of dysphagia diets, according to each patient's individual needs.

We have a nursery school at Burke, for employees' children. There is a program that brings the children into contact with the patients. This is wonderful to observe. The patients see them coloring, going to our greenhouse, and at play. Some of them seem to sparkle around children, which is wonderful therapy, especially at this time in their stroke. I have heard youngsters ask outright questions, such as "Why isn't your arm working?" And patients don't get angry and defensive, as they would if asked this by an impertinent adult. It is good to hear them giving the child an explanation, as best as possible.

We have a close working relationship with our physicians. We give them a report each morning, and are quickly informed of the medical opinions. They keep us on track, at all times. We also work closely with the dietician. Keeping some patients hydrated may be a problem. Many of them are afraid or unable to drink. Some can't take thin liquids, so we have to make sure they have thick liquids at their bedsides, at all times.

Our initial assessment of a patient includes nutritional needs. Skin care may become a big problem, but we try to heal that quickly. In this unit the patients are given showers, which is something they don't expect in a hospital. After having had only sponge baths, this is an uplifting experience.

Bowel and bladder problems are major concerns. Many patients go to live in nursing homes because of this. Families will gladly work with the patient on nearly everything else, but this area is particularly difficult. We try to train the patients, as well as their caregivers to overcome the inhibitions that continue to make this a predicament. It is usually more difficult for the patient's children to learn to help with bodily elimination needs.

With our bowel program we have learned that if we put a patient on a toilet, it is a lot better than using a bedpan. We have special chairs that facilitate wheeling the patient right over the toilet. That makes things a lot easier for the caregiver, as well.

We assess bladder control with a Doppler test. Without being invasive, this tells us how much urine is in the bladder. We try to establish two-hour schedules, but that is sometimes very difficult. The patient may want relief before the scheduled time, and we try to insist on holding it in, if possible. Naturally, we are not very popular, at these times. Retraining bladder control is very difficult and upsetting for the patient. Sometimes we are perceived as being insensitive or even cruel, because of this.

If possible, the patient is told to take his own medicine—under supervision, of course. This self-medication program also can be misinterpreted as laziness or uncaring, on the nurse's part. Actually, it takes us much longer to accomplish this, than it would to simply do it for the patient, each time. But nothing would be learned other than dependency.

Language deficits is probably one of the hardest problems to deal with. The patient can't communicate, and needs some way out of this dilemma. We try writing on small chalk boards, but this doesn't always work as well as would be desired. But the experienced professional begins to have some sixth sense of what the patient is thinking or feeling. Sometimes this proves to be extremely helpful.

We have to be constantly on the watch for possible accidents that can be caused by visual problems. A patient might burn himself on hot coffee, bump into walls, or get into a host of other problems.

It is often very hard for a family to understand that a patient's prestroke skills and abilities have nothing to do with his poststroke condition. It can seem that the stroke has left him unable to comprehend things, and that is usually very upsetting. They often get angry at the nurses. I would even say that some seem to hate us the first two weeks, or even longer. Our strict scheduling seems uncaring to them. They don't realize that, in a sense, we are like drill sergeants, working toward a very specific goal.

We try to encourage the use of day passes. It is good therapy to dress up in street clothes, again. Some of the best experiences we have noted is when female patients go to the hairdresser. They love it. Then they start putting on makeup, again, developing their outer self-image. It is so important to feel good about one's self. We train our nursing staff to see each patient as an individual, a person with feelings. Some nurses tend to focus on a patient's intake and output. That is good, but not nearly enough to satisfy the total human needs that can tend to be overlooked.

Family and other caregivers who sleep over, keeping the patient company, are often surprised at all the tiny details that must be attended to. If they are not taken care of immediately, they can get very upset. And that will upset the patient, as well. This is especially true, late at night, when minimal staff is on duty, and the daytime attention is not available. This kind of experience should be a vital part of the caregiver training.

In home care transition we try to bring in a family member or a hired caregiver. We train them for two or three weeks before discharge from the hospital. If there will be a visiting nurse service, we try to cooperate as fully as possible. We never stop caring for our patients. It is especially gratifying to hear from an occasional former patient, who calls up to say hello, tell us how he is doing, and perhaps ask a few questions.

Perhaps our greatest weakness in patient care comes from aides. Some people who come from foreign cultures sometimes can't perceive that things may not be right, from our Western cultural perspectives. The aide is often low-salaried, hired to do menial things that require understanding and training. Sometimes they say things to patients, that seem unkind. But from their cultural perspective, that would be acceptable. We are offering in-service training, focusing on patients' feelings and perspectives. It must also be kept in mind that sometimes stroke patients may scream at them, or even hit or punch them. The job isn't easy, and we have formed what we call "bitch groups," to vent the anger and help ease the situations.

Wherever possible, we try to teach our patients how to get on in social situations. It can be very embarrassing if one starts to cry–or even laugh–during an inappropriate public moment. We try to help our patients understand their stroke-related special problems, and live with them. Psychological counseling is very important to the well-being and total healing of the stroke patient.

One of the greatest rewards to our rehabilitation nurses is when former patients come back to visit. This is a big moment in their lives. They are always smiling, and dressed very well. Sometimes they are sporting a tan, and are eager to tell us about their trip to Florida, or wherever they went. But it is especially gratifying when they can say how they hated us, but now realize how much we actually did to help in their recovery. We try to have them visit some of our current patients, and that can make everybody feel good.

The job of a rehabilitation nurse in the stroke unit is as varied as it is responsible. We deal with human tragedy, but know that our special skills and temperament can make a great difference in the lives of stroke survivors and their return to the community.

Aphasia:
Rehabilitation and Recovery from Loss

Martha Taylor Sarno

All human beings experience losses in different ways from birth to death. Our reaction to loss, which encompasses denial, rage, and sorrow, seems to be fairly universal, though varied with respect to the sequence and duration. Aphasia can be characterized as a spectrum of losses which range from the privation of the ability to communicate through speech to an altered perception of familial, social and vocational roles. These are not single reactions, but very complicated processes that involve emotions and attempts to adjust to and cope with the loss–a mourning process. The process for the person with acquired aphasia is dynamic following the general outlines of stages proposed by many authors, notably Elizabeth Kubler-Ross, who characterized the stages of grief as attempts to overcome the feelings of loss.

Since earliest times human beings have searched for explanations of the origin of speech, particularly what is referred to as the power or the gift of speech and its remarkable efficiency as a code for communication. Indeed, the use of speech is an extraordinary and complex system which separates us from all other species. It is believed to be biologically determined, therefore, acquired–not learned, in the traditional sense. In all ways, it is a uniquely human behavior which plays a vital role in the human maturation process.

Martha Taylor Sarno, MA, MD (Hon), is Professor of Clinical Rehabilitation Medicine at the NYU School of Medicine, and Director of Speech-Language Pathology at the Howard A. Rusk Institute of Rehabilitation Medicine, NYU Medical Center. Dr. Sarno is the founder/president of the National Aphasia Association.

[Haworth co-indexing entry note]: "Aphasia: Rehabilitation and Recovery from Loss." Sarno, Martha Taylor. Co-published simultaneously in *Loss, Grief & Care* (The Haworth Press, Inc.) Vol. 8, No. 1/2, 1998, pp. 83-91; and: *After Stroke: Enhancing Quality of Life* (ed: Wallace Sife) The Haworth Press, Inc., 1998, pp. 83-91. Single or multiple copies of this article are available for a fee from The Haworth Document Delivery Service [1-800-342-9678, 9:00 a.m. - 5:00 p.m. (EST). E-mail address: getinfo@haworth.com].

83

The mechanisms which underlie the emergence of human communication are not well understood. Yet, children acquire speech and language skills without effort. Even in the most primitive societies, human beings have shared their experiences, ideas and feelings through speech. The use of speech for communication is universal, whereas not all human communities have systems of writing or reading.

To understand the complexity and diversity of human communication we must realize that even among unimpaired speakers, speech behavior has great variability. In fact, we employ hundreds of different sounds, each with varying characteristics, even within the same words, to transmit information. But listeners do not rely exclusively on information derived from the speech sounds alone, but also depend on contextual cues. These cues encompass all other aspects of communication and influence the extent to which a message can be communicated. These cues include the reason to communicate, the level of formality required by the communicator, and the degree of knowledge the participants have pertaining to the subject being communicated. For example, if the listener grasps the topic of conversation, and has previous knowledge regarding it, they are more likely to understand the communicator's message even without hearing all of the speech sounds.

Communicative interactions also depend on the neurologic specification of the timing and synchrony of both the motor speech system and the cognitive-semantic system. Nonverbal pragmatic behaviors such as "turn taking," gestures and pantomime, also contribute to the communication interaction. Communication behavior, therefore, includes automatic speech, vocabulary, melodic intonation, word stress, grammar, and the quality of voice which differentiate one speaker from another. As the distinguished neurologist, MacDonald Chritchley once said, "Each person's manner of using language is very individual and personal and never altogether shared with the rest of the community" (Critchley, 1970). Indeed, speech behavior is central to a person's identity and personality.

Since aphasia strikes at the very heart of personhood, it is no wonder that its onset has a profoundly negative effect on a person's sense of self. Aphasia represents a loss of a part of the self, a changed identity. Many authors describe the self as dependent on and defined through social interaction. Abe Raskin addressed his new identity as a person with aphasia when he wrote, "It's difficult to convey the depths of my emotional solitude. I did not feel like Abe Raskin. I now had a new self, a person who no longer could use words with mastery. Privately, I could do nothing but cry, but with the tears came feelings of anxiety and depression. I wavered between feelings of melancholy and hope" (Raskin, 1992). It has been said that the person with aphasia mourns the loss of self in terms of a loss of identity. Family and caregivers also participate in the need to find a new identity, a new post-stroke self.

Certain attitudes about speech function set aphasia apart as a disability which dehumanizes and isolates the individual. For centuries speechlessness was referred to as "dumb," implying diminished mental competence. Though the term "deaf and dumb" is unacceptable in contemporary society, the attitude apparently persists. Only a few years ago, a book which dealt with the trial of an individual who was congenitally deaf and unable to produce intelligible speech was titled *Dummy*. This coupled with the prevailing view of the elderly as second class citizens, transmits a demeaning minority status to the older aphasic patient. Little wonder that many with acquired aphasia feel weak, insignificant, and very unimportant.

An additional disadvantage for people with aphasia, even among disabled peers, is the invisible aspect of the disability. It is easy to be aware of and helpful toward someone who is blind, paralyzed, or missing a limb. But there are no signals to tell us that a person with aphasia is in our midst. This fact may enhance the perception that someone with aphasia is indeed "dumb," deranged or even psychotic. One person with mild aphasia whose physical disability had resolved, said, "I wish my arm was open and bleeding so that people could see that something is wrong." The person with aphasia has to live with both the reality of the condition and the failure of society to be aware of and acknowledge the communication impairment. The presence of aphasia interferes with the ability to initiate and maintain personal relationships, one of the most basic elements in our sense of self and the feeling of belonging to the larger human community (Sarno, 1986).

In a survey conducted by the National Aphasia Association in 1988, seventy-five percent of the respondents said that they believe that people avoided them because of their communication difficulties. Having to cope with being socially different, the loss of self esteem and possible depression in the face of suddenly impaired communication, renders the person with aphasia socially handicapped. One of the most devastating results of aphasia is the inability to share experiences with others. A contributing factor to this inability is the discomfort that many normal speakers feel when they deal with people who can't communicate very well. This may lead to a withdrawal of outside support which surfaces as an inability to take part in healing conversation–a behavior which is thought to allow individuals to adjust to emotional trauma. Aphasia then, is a ruthless condition as it interferes with the crucial vehicle of its own treatment.

Living with aphasia is not an easy process. It is most successful when individuals and those closest to them can grieve their losses while developing, accepting and creating a new "self." The family unit which suffers in a state of disequilibrium, when one of its members acquires aphasia, is at high risk for negative reactions. Some experience severe psychosocial alterations in their everyday lives and cannot cope with the future. Internal family dynamics, including decreased social activity, role reversal and additional work and responsibility directly related to the individual with aphasia, increase the tension. Family members may become anxious, angry, feel out of control and overwhelmed. This situation can lead to a vicious cycle of loneliness, frustration and withdrawal from society, with resulting social isolation. A confounding point is the deliberation of whether or not these feelings existed in the pre-stroke state, and are simply magnified by the acquired disability.

Some of these issues may have been overlooked in aphasia rehabilitation because, historically, the field of medicine has made high-tech acute care issues its primary concern. Also, the chronic nature of aphasia causes it to lack the visibility and fascination of the high-tech dramas that are played out in the acute care setting. A predominating biomedical approach leaves little room to address the social-psychological and behavioral dimensions of illness. The traditional medical model, limited to identifying the characteristics of diseases, their etiologies, pathology, and manifestations, is still the model of choice. Acute restorative care in the medical model is accomplished through clinical procedures like surgery and drugs, and limits its definition of the pathology almost entirely to patients' physical, rather than psychological and social dimensions. In the traditional model it is assumed that if the patient complies with the physician's orders he or she will be cured. Since aphasia is usually a long-term, chronic disability, practitioners should aspire beyond the medical model and incorporate an understanding of the inevitable psychological and social consequences.

The contrasting philosophies of health care, acute care and rehabilitation or restorative care, become apparent when parameters such as goalsetting are examined. In traditional medicine, goals are determined almost entirely by the physician, who is the ultimate authority. In a field like rehabilitation medicine, on the other hand, the patient, family and team set the goals together, often with the rehabilitation medicine physician managing the negotiation of the treatment goals.

People with aphasia share a fear with others who are chronically ill–of being permanently incapacitated, dependent, and perhaps institutionalized. This contemplation is so frightening that it is often denied in order to preserve any semblance of hope. However, denial can be a constructive and useful tool, since it allows patients and families to borrow time while coming to terms with reality and recovery. In many cases the use of denial as a defense mechanism may relate to the way in which a person with aphasia had coped with adversity before acquiring aphasia.

Emotional reactions to aphasia are undoubtedly influenced by pre-morbid personality and values, which tend to become exaggerated by the pre-morbid view the person had of impairment, disability, and handicap. Premorbid conceptions may also influence how people with aphasia view themselves in an altered disabled state. Rehabilitation can be viewed as the process of helping an individual become a new self in order to successfully reintegrate into society. Successful rehabilitation, according to Maslow (1968), is achieved when the patient's focus on mere survival shifts to a focus on self-actualization. Yet, the disabled person often has a reduced drive for self-actualization, and rehabilitation goals must take this into account or all efforts may fail. Maslow points out a fundamental relationship between the self concept and the rehabilitation process. He describes that the latter necessitates redefining the quality of life in an altered state, perhaps even adopting a new philosophy of life (Maslow, 1968). Enlisting one's inner resources to do this, be they of spirit, faith, philosophy, or ego strength, is not often in concert with the rehabilitation medicine physician managing the negotiation of the treatment goals. Enlisting one's inner resources to do this, be they of spirit, faith, philosophy, or ego strength, is not always possible. It does not come easily to those whose primary life values depended on material rather than aesthetic fulfillment. Interestingly, it is not unusual to hear a person who acquired aphasia report that aphasia caused them to reevaluate and redefine their lives, philosophy, values, and find a more fulfilling way of life.

A remarkable example of this is that of Joseph Chaikin, the well-known dramatist, playwright, actor, and director, who acquired aphasia. He continues to work in the theater actively, except that now, the theater is a vehicle for the expression of his pain as a person with aphasia. For several years, Chaikin could only stutter the word, "yes," and he continues to have very severe deficits in comprehension and speech production. But he is able through gesture and a limited vocabulary to carry on an extraordinarily active life in the theater. Chaikin reports that in some ways he finds his new "self" more fulfilling and likable than his old "self." He describes, in some of his poetry and readings, how much he has learned about life from the experience of aphasia which has strengthened him. Joseph Chaikin is an inspiring example of someone who has recreated himself.

The abrupt onset of aphasia adds a dimension, and can delay adaptation for some. This is especially true when the caregiver is elderly and already struggling to cope with the realities and limitations imposed by aging. In addition to problems within the family unit, there is the larger issue of society's response. The aphasia community and the health professionals who work with them are faced with an enormous educational challenge which must be met, if those with aphasia are to live in a society which facilitates and fosters community reintegration for individuals with chronic disabilities.

It is mistakenly assumed that family adjustments improve naturally, with time. Yet in one study, a third of stroke patients' families described themselves as maladjusted two to five years post-onset. Clearly, families of people with aphasia are under considerable stress, due to the sudden and severe disruption in family life. The abrupt intrusion of aphasia, its interference with freeflowing verbal exchange, unpredictable course, and inevitable impact on the family's sources of gratification, represents a major shift in the family life cycle. In one study, spouses of patients with aphasia evidenced significantly poorer rapport and overall social adjustment, when compared to spouses of non-aphasic stroke patients (Kinsella and Duffy, 1979). Aphasia also impairs the shared social and leisure life so important for the family unit. Understandably, communication is often reported as a severe problem in the marriages of both aphasic and non-aphasic stroke patients. Relatives report a feeling of loss in dealing with the person with aphasia and the feeling that the person is no longer there.

Some family members harbor unreasonably high expectations for the individual's recovery and function. Studies confirm that there may be a natural tendency to minimize the patient's communication impairment. Optimism on the part of patients and relatives is often explained as a lack of sufficient knowledge about aphasia. More often than not, the person with aphasia does not meet the unrealistic recovery expectations, and in time the patient and family grow increasingly frustrated, sometimes enraged.

The term *recovery* is open to a wide range of interpretations by the patient, family and health professionals. Most patients do not consider themselves recovered unless they have returned fully to previous levels of communication competence. Recovery, after all, is a subjective perception, and should not be confused with an objective evaluation of communication skills. The final evaluation of outcome must be measured by the patient's perception of his/her quality of life.

Many ethical and moral dilemmas come into play in the clinical management of people with aphasia. These include such issues as patient selection, patient autonomy, the determination of rehabilitation regimens, the setting of goals, and how and when treatment will be terminated. A unique feature of rehabilitation services in the United States is the fact that they are not an "entitlement" and practitioners choose their patients. As a result of limited rehabilitation resources and the patient selection process, those who receive rehabilitation services tend to be more educated, affluent and assertive. Those from less privileged circumstances may require additional rehabilitation resources in order to achieve rehabilitation goals.

An individual's access to rehabilitation services is influenced by the person's presumed potential for recovery potential, ability to pay for treatment, the anticipated burden the individual will place on the rehabilitation team, and the amount of available outside support which the patient may be expected to receive. As a primary criterion in patient selection, some agencies and third party payers use potential to resume employment following rehabilitation. Thus, they give younger patients priority over older patients.

As a result, there is a prevailing misconception that recovery in the person with aphasia takes place only in the first six months post-stroke. A large number of patients are disqualified from receiving services after the early post-acute period. Unfortunately, the majority of patients are not told the reason they are rejected from participation, and patients sometimes interpret the rejection as an indication of a negative prognosis. Patients who have been excluded from aphasia rehabilitation services may hold this view even two and three years after a stroke. Furthermore, the feeling often translates itself into a belief on the part of people with aphasia that they were not worthy of treatment.

In addition to limitations imposed by the criteria employed in selecting patients to receive rehabilitation services, other serious ethical-moral questions emerge. For example, regarding the potential to benefit criterion, in aphasia rehabilitation the definition of benefit may be defined in different ways. It can relate to an increased rate of speech production, greater comprehension and expressive skills, or the ability to be independent. But the rehabilitation process was not created to select and endorse a single cure, inherent in the acute medical model. Rather, rehabilitation addresses restoration of function and improvement in the patient's quality of life.

The ethical-moral issues raised by these practices are significant. Future efforts need to be geared toward offering services to all patients, albeit in different forms, on a continuous basis, at the optimum times for improvement of communication skills. The times when the person can benefit from intervention vary greatly and depend on many factors, beginning with the type, severity, and time since the onset of aphasia.

Many individuals with aphasia, whether involved in a clinical treatment or research program, also harbor the idea that by being selected there is an implied promise of improvement (i.e., recovery). In the clinical area, the promise of benefit is implied in the "halo" effect, the notion that our high-tech society can overcome any adversity, including complete recovery from aphasia.

The open-ended nature of the aphasia rehabilitation process poses important dilemmas, and requires negotiation among the principal characters in the rehabilitation scenario. This includes the patient, family, physician, third party payer, and members of the rehabilitation team. Negotiation can be influenced by the degree of power each has at different stages in the rehabilitation process. How to control for this is a major challenge.

The termination of rehabilitation for the person with aphasia presents another moral quandary. When and how should it take place, whose standards and values should guide those decisions, and where should rehabilitation end and educational/social agency care begin? Can the termination of speech therapy be considered the equivalent of abandonment in the rehabilitation context (Sarno, 1993 & 1986)? Although precise data are not available it is generally believed that the population of people with aphasia who might benefit from access to speech pathology services in the United States far exceeds the number who are receiving treatment.

For most, aphasia therapy must be intensive, comprehensive, and of a long duration. The cost of private therapy is often prohibitive, and the availability of public funds severely limited. Restricted reimbursements for services makes aphasia rehabilitation unattainable for most. It is unlikely that this situation is going to improve in the immediate future unless there is an increase in the number of studies which support the efficacy of aphasia rehabilitation, and document the psycho-social impact of the disorder, thereby supporting the need for clinical management over long periods of time. Another no less important obstacle is the inadequate number of speech and language pathologists who have special interest and expertise in aphasia.

The cure-oriented, high-tech, basis for much current medical practice and health care policy does not address the quality of life needs of the chronically ill, and is unresponsive to the meaning and impact of aphasia on the individual, community and society. Chronic disabilities like aphasia are a moral challenge because they force us to confront the question of "how a good society should accommodate the expectable, but always unexpected misfortunes occur in everyone's life" (Jennings et al., 1988). Through the provision of care and social support to people with chronic disabilities, those of us who are temporarily well and able-bodied acknowledge the bonds among human beings, our universal frailty and the uncertainty of the human condition. The ethical-moral issues associated with aphasia epitomize the challenges posed by chronic disability.

AUTHOR NOTE

This article is an adaptation of invited papers presented at the Fifth International Aphasia Rehabilitation Conference, Zurich, 1992, and the Sixth International Aphasia Rehabilitation Conference, Aalborg, Denmark, 1994 and the paper "Aphasia rehabilitation: Psychosocial and ethical considerations," *Aphasiology*, 1993, vol. 7, no. 4, 321-334.

Preparation of this paper was supported in part by the National Institute of Deafness and Other Communication Disorders (NIDCD) grant RO1NS25367-01A1 (of which the author is Principal Investigator) and the National Institute of Disability and Rehabilitation Research (NIDRR) grant G00830000.

REFERENCES

Critchley, M. *Aphasiology and Other Aspects of Language.* London: Edward Arnold, 1970.

Jennings, B., Callahan, D. and Caplan, A.L. "Ethical Challenges of Chronic Illness." A Hastings Center Report (Feb./Mar.), Briarcliff Manor, NY, 1988.

Kinsella, G.J. and Duffy, F.D. "Psychosocial Readjustment in the Spouses of Aphasic Patients." *Scandinavian Journal of Rehabilitation Medicine, 11,* 129-132, 1979.

Maslow, A.H. *Toward a Psychology of Being.* Van Nostrand, Princeton, NJ, 1968.

Raskin, A.H., "The Words I Lost." *New York Times*, Sept. 19th, p. 19, 1992.

Sarno, M.T. *The Silent Minority: The Patient with Aphasia.* Fifth Annual James C. Hemphill Lecture, Rehabilitation Institute of Chicago, September 24, 1986. Published by the Rehabilitation Institute of Chicago, 1986.

Sarno, M.T. "Aphasia Rehabilitation: Psychosocial and Ethical Considerations," *7,* 321-334, 1993.

Sarno, M.T. "Quality of Life in Aphasia in the First Year Post Stroke." *Aphasiology,* 1995.

Dysphagia:
Swallowing Disorders Following a Stroke

Joyce Bores

As a vital member of the stroke team, the speech pathologist is sometimes perceived as a specialist limited to problems related to speech production. But dysphagia is her concern, as well. About one out of every three stroke patients demonstrates some swallowing disorder, which could become life-threatening, if appropriate therapy is not given early in the recovery process (Veis, Logemann, 1985).

Aside from the threat of choking or respiratory distress, the mechanics of eating may become a difficult and laborious task. The dysphagic individual may be robbed of the pleasure that food may have held, before the onset of the stroke. It is the challenge of the speech pathologist to help improve the safety and efficiency of the stroke patient's swallowing function, as well as help him regain optimum nutrition.

Dysphagia can result from both cortical lesions and subcortical brain stem lesions. But there has not been any clear association between specific types of dysphagia and the site of lesions. Dysphagia is classified in three stages: the oral stage, the pharyngal stage, and the esophageal stage. In the oral stage, food is first received into the mouth. The lips are closed, and one chews and manipulates the food, forming it into a cohesive bolus, getting it ready to transfer to the throat. Then the tongue will elevate and move posteriorly, to propel the food into the pharynx.

In the pharyngal stage, the pharyngeal swallow is triggered. There is some controversy, however, about at exactly what point this takes place. In

Joyce Bores, MS, CCC, is affiliated with the Kessler Institute for Rehabilitation, Inc. at Saddle Brook, NJ.

[Haworth co-indexing entry note]: "Dysphagia: Swallowing Disorders Following a Stroke." Bores, Joyce. Co-published simultaneously in *Loss, Grief & Care* (The Haworth Press, Inc.) Vol. 8, No. 1/2, 1998, pp. 93-98; and: *After Stroke: Enhancing Quality of Life* (ed: Wallace Sife) The Haworth Press, Inc., 1998, pp. 93-98. Single or multiple copies of this article are available for a fee from The Haworth Document Delivery Service [1-800-342-9678, 9:00 a.m. - 5:00 p.m. (EST). E-mail address: getinfo@haworth.com].

the back of the mouth, there is the fossa arch that was traditionally thought of as the place where the swallow is begun. However, others have found that the swallow may start at the vallecula, just superior to the epiglottis in the hypopharynx.

Next, the soft palate elevates as it retracts, closing off the velopharyngeal port. Then food is squeezed through by the pharyngeal muscles. The larynx elevates, pulls forward and is closed. The vocal cords close off the airway to protect it. The cricopharyngeal sphincter opening then relaxes for passage of food to the esophagus.

The esophageal stage begins at this point. The esophageal muscles squeeze the food down to the lower esophagus (the gastroesophageal junctura, or opening to the stomach). This is very highly coordinated, well-sequenced series of movements.

The evaluation of dysphagia is most often accomplished by a multi-disciplined team. It involves a number of professionals, including physicians such as neurologists, otolaryngologists, physiatrists and gastroenterologists—as well as many therapists, speech and language pathologists, and nurses. There is a wide range of health care professionals who work with patients who have swallowing problems.

The role of the speech pathologist is not only as an integral part of an evaluation team, but one which carries out the recommended treatment for dysphagia. This includes patient/family education and training. However, we cannot treat these patients alone. The exchange of information from all members of the team serves to aid in better treatment of the patient, medically and therapeutically. We need to consider medical histories and evaluations from physicians, other health care professionals, as well as subjective reports from patients—in making appropriate decisions for treatment and referrals.

One of the responsibilities of the speech pathologist is to perform the bedside evaluation. At first, the speech language pathologist will make observations about cognitive and perceptual abilities. The occupational therapist will also have input to this. He or she will pay particular attention to the patient's alertness level, awareness of difficulties, attention and concentration, and will evaluate comprehension, memory, visual perception and eye-hand coordination for feeding.

The speech pathologist will then perform an oral motor assessment, evaluating the strength, movement and sensation of the swallow mechanism. He will examine the muscles in the face, jaw, teeth (are they adequate for chewing?) lips, tongue, and the soft palate. He will also examine for a gag reflex. Studies have shown that there is a high correlation between this and the prevalence of aspiration in people recovering from a stroke. Aspiration means that food or liquid is taken into the airway, and can eventually end up in the lungs. This may cause infection and pneumonia, and is one of the reasons we are so concerned with swallowing problems.

Some other procedures a speech pathologist will perform during a bedside exam may begin with a laryngeal function assessment. At this time we look at laryngeal elevation by palpating the swallow. The speech pathologist will put her finger on the bone at the thyroid notch, below the larynx, ask the patient to swallow, and then feel what happens. She will also listen to see if there are unusual sounds, while looking for an elevation of the larynx and a pulling forward. Then the patient is asked to cough voluntarily. The cough is our protective reflex. If a foreign object enters the airway, or the patient does not have an adequate cough, he may not be able to protect his airway from aspiration.

Throat clearing is another protective mechanism which we assess. Then a gross assessment of phonation is made. The speech pathologist will ask the patient to phonate, make "ah" and "ooh" sounds. This examines laryngeal functioning for closing off the airway, which is also a function of the vocal chords. We also rely upon the expertise of the otolaryngologist who performs a more extensive evaluation of laryngeal function.

We observe the respiratory mechanism, and its effects on swallowing, using a stethoscope. Chronic obstructive pulmonary disease (COPD) results in shortness of breath and loss of coordinated swallowing with breathing. The patient needs to take breaths so quickly that he can't complete a swallow before he has to breathe, again. Thus, patients may end up inspiring food.

If the patient's mechanism appears adequate enough to tolerate ingestion, the speech pathologist will then assess with food, and examine the patient's posture. Can he control his body and head, in order to self-feed? Does he have the ability to manipulate the food, move it in the mouth and swallow? The examiner will also discover a little bit about the esophageal function, by asking the patient if he has any problem with heartburn. Of course, if a patient should vomit during the exam, then it is evident that there is a problem.

After dysphagia has been identified, the next step is to further evaluate the videofluoroscopic swallowing study. This is dynamic radiographic evaluation of swallowing, during which the patient is positioned upright. It examines the oral cavity, pharynx, larynx and the esophagus, in both lateral and anterior to posterior plains. It gives us vital information in order to manage the swallowing problems. It identifies motility difficulties in the oral pharyngal and esophageal stages. It assesses oral and pharyngal transit time, and assesses aspiration–why and when it occurs. It helps determine treatment strategies that may be effective in helping the patient improve his swallowing. It can help determine recommendations for diet. We do this exam with varying textures of food and liquids, and mix it with bariums so it may be viewed in the fluoroscopic image.

Disorders of swallowing may occur in the oral stage, where rapid ingestion may result in impaired sequencing between oral transit and airway closure. Also, an individual can lose control of the bolus, because of disorganized or weak tongue movements. This then prematurely spills to the throat, and may enter the unprotected airway. In the oral stage there can be a complete disassociation between oral transit and the initiation of the pharyngeal stage.

Disorders of this stage may occur if initiation of the swallow is delayed or weak. Bolus material can spill into the airway. Also, if there is incomplete laryngeal elevation or if the muscles of the pharynx are not strong enough to push the food through quickly, aspiration may occur during the swallow. This may also occur after the swallow, because of residue pooled in the throat, due to weakness or paralysis of the throat muscles.

Aspiration can also result from esophageal dysfunction such as reflux, spasm, diverticulum, stricture or achalasia. Food material may be diverted upward from the esophagus into the pharynx, where it can be aspirated.

It is important to establish goals, early on. We want optimal means of nutrition for a patient, and need to learn which foods are going to be appealing to him. It is easy to decide to give a patient pureed food, but will he really accept it? Not necessarily. And, that's one of the challenges in treating these difficulties. We want to facilitate a safe pattern of eating and drinking so the patient doesn't develop pneumonia.

We will intervene with patients in NPO status, who are not getting food by mouth. They may be fed with a nasogastric tube or gastrostomy. The swallowing is treated indirectly via oral motor exercise and stimulation. We might practice therapeutic maneuvers with them, using their saliva only. We may also initiate therapeutic feedings with them, giving them very small amounts of food, by mouth.

With those who can eat, we might modify diet textures. Liquids may need to be thickened. Many patients don't like thick liquids, but it may be the safest way to drink, at least initially when they are first recovering. It may also be necessary to change the texture to make it easier to swallow.

We teach different postures, such as neck flexion, widening an area in the throat to enhance airway protection, and also the clearing of residual food materials. Neck rotation, turning the head to the paralyzed side, closes the paralyzed side so the strong side does all the work.

Head extension entails putting the head a little bit back, to help gravity guide food from the mouth and down. This is especially helpful if patients are having significant oral transit difficulties. However, this is never done with patients who aspirate.

Thermal stimulation is done by taking a cold object, such as a dental mirror, and stimulating the area in the back of the mouth where the swallow is thought to be initiated. Supra glottic swallow is a therapeutic maneuver in which you ask a patient to hold his breath and bear down, swallow, cough and swallow again. You are making him close off the airway, and expel any food materials at the top of the airway, after the swallow. Then he is to swallow again, to get clear those residuals.

Mendelssohn's Maneuver helps to elevate the larynx and remove food materials from the pharynx. This increases motility of food through the pharynx. We may ask patients to alternate their liquids and solids while they are eating, slow down while they eat, or take small amounts instead of big ones.

Finally, we provide education to the family or caregiver, reviewing the results of the evaluation. It is important to explain what the symptoms mean, and discuss and demonstrate treatment strategies, as well as the need for careful follow-up.

This job of the SLP is to effectively manage the poststroke life-threatening aspects of dysphagia. The therapy is slow and meticulous, but the rewards to the patient are also rewards to the speech therapist, who provides this vital and lesser-known service.

SUGGESTED READING

Alberts, M. J. et al. (1992). "Aspiration After Stroke: Lesion Analysis by Brain MRI." *Dysphagia,* 7, 170-173.

Bastian, R. W. (1991). "Videoendoscopic Evaluation of Patients with Dysphagia: An Adjunct to Modified Barium Swallow." *Otolaryngol Head Neck Surgery,* 104 (3)338-150.

Buchholz, D. (1987). "Neurological Evaluation of Dysphagia." *Dysphagia,* 1:187-192.

Butcher, R. B. (1982). "Treatment of Chronic Aspiration as a Complication of Cerebrovascular Accident." *Laryngoscope,* 92: 681-685.

Gordon, C., Hewer, R. L., Wade, D. T. (1987). "Dysphagia in Acute Stroke." *British Med. Jour.,* 295: 411-414.

Grohar, M. E. and Bukatman, R. (1986). "The Prevalence of Swallowing Disorders in Two Teaching Hospitals." *Dysphagia,* 1: 3-6.

Homer, J., Massay, E. W. (1988). "Silent Aspiration Following Stroke." *Neurology,* 38: 317-319.

Homer, J. (1991). "Dysphagia in Neurologic Disease" Presentation at Swallowing and Swallowing Disorders: From Clinic to Laboratory,–a conference at Northwestern Univ., Evanston, IL.

Langmore, S. E., Logemann, J. A. (1991). "After the Clinical Bedside Swallowing Examination: What Next?" *American Journal of Speech-Language Pathology*, 1: 13-20.

Langmore, S. E., Schatz, K., Olsen, N. (1988). "Fiberoptic Endoscopic Examination of Swallowing Safety: A New Procedure." *Dysphagia*, 2: 216-219.

Langmore, S. E. (1991). "Managing the Complications of Aspiration in Dysphagic Adults." In Sonies, B. C. (ed.), *Seminars in Speech and Language*, 12(3), 199-207. NY, Thieme Med. Pub.

Sonies, B. C. (1991). "Instrumental Procedures for Dysphagia Diagnosis." *Seminars in Speech and Language*, 12, (3): 199-207.

Veis, S. L., Logemann, J. A. (1985). "Swallowing Disorders in Persons with Cerebrovascular Accident." *Arch. Phys. Med. Rehab.*, 66: 372-375.

Management
of the Communicatively Challenged Adult
After Stroke:
Partners in Rehabilitation

Joyce Bores

In addition to dysphagia, there are many possible negative effects, that may result from a stroke. This can also include impairments in speech and language production and use, comprehension and underlying cognitive processes such as memory, attention/concentration, reasoning and executive function. Changes in behavior can also affect the appropriateness of communication. The impact of such deficits upon daily life can be devastating to both stroke victim as well as his/her family. Adjustments must be made not only to the communication impairments but to long term changes in the social, financial and emotional structure of the family (Marquardt, 1982).

If we are to consider the quality of life after stroke, effective management of the communicatively challenged adult is essential in the rehabilitation process. This has been defined by Goldberg (1974) as the process of restoring a handicapped person if not to the level of function and social position which he had achieved before the onset of illness then at least to a situation in which he/she can make best use of residual capacities within as normal as possible a social context. If this is to be achieved, inclusion of the family or caregiver as partner in treatment can help to facilitate adapta-

Joyce Bores, MS, CCC, is affiliated with the Kessler Institute for Rehabilitation, Inc. at Saddle Brook, NJ.

[Haworth co-indexing entry note]: "Management of the Communicatively Challenged Adult After Stroke: Partners in Rehabilitation." Bores, Joyce. Co-published simultaneously in *Loss, Grief & Care* (The Haworth Press, Inc.) Vol. 8, No. 1/2, 1998, pp. 99-101; and: *After Stroke: Enhancing Quality of Life* (ed: Wallace Sife) The Haworth Press, Inc., 1998, pp. 99-101. Single or multiple copies of this article are available for a fee from The Haworth Document Delivery Service [1-800-342-9678, 9:00 a.m. - 5:00 p.m. (EST). E-mail address: getinfo@haworth.com].

99

tion to changes in communication abilities. However, these individuals must have realistic expectations of their loved ones. Family education, training and counseling are an essential component of speech therapy in the rehabilitation process.

The role of the speech/language pathologist is as demanding as it is varied. Effective treatment of speech and language impairment begins with a comprehensive assessment of an individual's abilities and disabilities, as well as needs relative to his/her lifestyle. The speech pathologist also will administer diagnostic tests, and informally observe communication behaviors both in clinical and as natural settings as possible. An interview with family members is also recommended. Then, treatment may be planned. It should include clear long and short term objectives, agreed upon by all partners in care. This includes the speech pathologist, her client, and the family, as well.

In treating communication impairment, the role of the speech pathologist therefore includes:

1. Directing treatment toward specified disordered communicative processes.
2. Reducing environmental demands and increasing environmental opportunity for communication.
3. Providing information and support (Marquardt, 1982).

According to Mulhall (1988), aphasic individuals can develop an over-dependency on the speech/language pathologist as communicative partner. That generally results from dramatically increased effectiveness or efficiency of communicative interactions with this person. It therefore behooves the speech/language pathologist to model these skills with the whole family, as part of the treatment regimen.

Establishing rapport with the caregivers paves the opportunity for discussion and problem solving. It is possible that they may underestimate or even overestimate the communicative and cognitive abilities of the stroke survivor. The underestimating family may tend to be overprotective, even to the point of discouraging their loved one from trying activities. They often speak and make decisions for him, without even having involved him in any prior discussion.

On the other hand, the overestimating family usually has other unrealistic or inaccurate expectations that may frustrate or exhaust their loved one. Almost without exception, he will feel misunderstood. In either case, the family may be programming the stroke survivor for failure, without realizing the potentially destructive effects of their misapplied loving care. His already fragile feelings of self-worth are easily diminished or even extinguished. All too often these people feel victimized, defeated and inferior, lacking confidence and hope. As a result, they may completely withdraw from communication and interaction with everyone around them.

The speech/language pathologist provides education regarding the client's specific communication impairment and its remediation. This professional will give individualized guidance and training, in adjusting the communicative demands placed upon the patient. In structuring the environment for optimal communicative function, she will develop use of compensatory strategies by the client as well as the family, and provide practice in functional situations. This may be accomplished via role playing or community visits. Sometimes alternative methods, such as communication boards or books are needed.

Because of the personal nature of their work, speech/language pathologists are often privy to patient and family adjustment issues. Thus, they are in an excellent position to refer their clients to other professionals such as psychologists or social workers.

Lastly, the speech/language pathologist may provide information regarding stroke clubs, aphasia groups, caregiver support groups and supportive organizations such as the National Stroke Association and the National Aphasia Association. Her efforts to educate, provide information, support and referral are ongoing, throughout the rehabilitation partnership with the client and family.

There is a great sense of accomplishment in helping the survivor of stroke regain and develop a positive quality of life and self-image. The rewards, though not so tangible, are very meaningful to the person who becomes a professional, trained and dedicated to help others.

SUGGESTED READING

Broida, H., *Coping With Stroke.* College Hill Press, 1979.

Goldberg, D., *Principles of Rehabilitation Comprehensive Psychiatry,* 15, 237-249 (1974).

Gordon, W. A., *Advances in Stroke Rehabilitation.* Andover Medical Publishers, 1993.

Marquardt, T. P., *Acquired Neurogenic Disorders,* Prentice Hall, 1992.

Mulhall, D., "The Management of the Aphasic Patient." Rose, Whutr, Wyke, *Aphasia,* Chapter 20, Whurr Publishers Limited, 1988.

The Speech/Language Pathologist: Bridging the Communication Gap

Karen Dikeman
Marta Kazandjian

"SLP: Bridging the Communication Gap" is a theme which we have emphasized in several of our presentations at conferences. For speech clinicians, the title illustrates how we view our role in helping the communicatively impaired person who has experienced a stroke. The SLP addresses a variety of concerns stemming from a stroke, so our work extends beyond the traditional concept of the therapist who works on speech drills in a standard treatment room. To successfully help an individual, following a stroke, the SLP must also be a counselor and educator, resource person and patient advocate. The SLP determines how to help the person with a communication disorder, experienced after a stroke. She serves as a member of a professional therapeutic team, which involves above all, the individual and family who have experienced the stroke.

Aphasia is a language disorder. It is most usually a result of a left hemisphere lesion in the brain, which affects normal linguistic functioning. Aphasia is considered a language problem because it affects the ability to recognize and manipulate the symbols (sounds and letters) upon which language is based. It can be differentiated from cognitive-linguistic

Karen Dikeman, MA, CCC-SLP and Marta Kazandjian, MA, CCC-SLP, are Speech/Language Pathologists at Silvercrest Extended Care Facility and Long Beach Medical Center, NY. They are clinicians, presenters and authors in the diagnosis and treatment of the neurologically impaired, including the tracheostomized and ventilator-dependent individual. They have co-authored and presented extensively in this field.

[Haworth co-indexing entry note]: "The Speech/Language Pathologist: Bridging the Communication Gap." Dikeman, Karen, and Marta Kazandjian. Co-published simultaneously in *Loss, Grief & Care* (The Haworth Press, Inc.) Vol. 8, No. 1/2, 1998, pp. 103-108; and: *After Stroke: Enhancing Quality of Life* (ed: Wallace Sife) The Haworth Press, Inc., 1998, pp. 103-108. Single or multiple copies of this article are available for a fee from The Haworth Document Delivery Service [1-800-342-9678, 9:00 a.m. - 5:00 p.m. (EST). E-mail address: getinfo@haworth.com].

impairment associated with right hemisphere dysfunction or from diffuse neurological damage. Aphasic language impairment can range from profound to mild, but is consistently devastating in its effects. Aphasia impacts upon all areas of language: expression, understanding, reading, writing and even gesture.

Reports from individuals with mild aphasia, or from those who have recovered from a severe language deficit, speak of frustration and confusion, of hearing their own words sound foreign in their ears, of opening their mouths to ask for a drink of water and saying something that isn't even close, or of not even being able to write their own names.

The SLP who works with the stroke survivor with aphasia must know not only the type and severity of the language deficit, but the person's preferred communication style, communication partners and communication environment. She must understand what is important to this person.

We currently work with a woman in her early 40's. She is already several years post a devastating stroke, although her physical appearance does not provide any indication that she had any neurological involvement. She is married with two teenage children. What situations are important to her? This was as vital an issue during our assessment as was determining her level of reading comprehension, or how accurately she spelled words. Once we understood what was important in her life we developed a communication book and wallet card for her, which is still evolving today. It enabled her to write down all the important components involved in giving her daughter a college graduation party, and plan a family vacation. During the appropriate family discussion, out came her book from which she read aloud, joining in with much effort. This returned to her an element of participation and control in family life, which as a wife and mother, she sorely missed. This is not to say, of course, that there were and are not periods of being angry at children who are too impatient to allow her to slowly read her ideas. Nor does it imply that there is no frustration at not being able to spontaneously join in a simple conversation.

Another diagnosis commonly experienced after a stroke is dysarthria. This speech disorder impacts on the strength and accuracy of the speech musculature, so that the utterance sounds distorted and slurred, perhaps too loud or too soft in varying degrees. Dysphonia is another term, referring specifically to impairment of voice. Although the person with dysarthria or dysphonia may be well able to understand and produce complex sentences, his communicative exchanges may be unsuccessful because his speech is so difficult to understand. Speech intelligibility is only a particular area the SLP must focus on when assessing the person with dysarthria.

A secondary characteristic is often noticed; weakness of the oral mechanism also impacts upon the simple ability to control one's own saliva.

Drooling is a common symptom and source of great concern for many of our patients. We have had many patients who have shared with us their embarrassment and their subsequent reluctance to join social events, because of their drooling. The devastating effects of the stroke not only disrupt the person's ability to communicate but impact on the survivor's image of self. Self esteem can also be dealt a blow when the stroke survivor looks into a mirror and sees a face that is twisted with a pronounced facial droop. One of our patients was attempting to complete some facial exercises we had prescribed, and looked in a mirror for the first time, after her stroke. She was unable to complete her treatment session because, until then, she had not been aware of her facial droop. She was shocked, and our role quickly switched from therapist to counselor, as we began to listen and empathize with her emotional distress.

The stroke survivor may have an additional difficulty with dysphagia, or swallowing impairment. Because of the similar neuromuscular involvement, dysphagia and dysarthria are often associated. In addition to these difficulties, the dysphagic person may face a life-threatening impairment, which impacts upon the simple ability to take food and liquid by mouth. Those stroke survivors who have the most severe dysphagic impairment must at times rely on an alternate feeding method, such as a nasal or gastric feeding tube. Food and engaging in mealtime activity, normally is one of our greatest pleasures and often the center of our social and family lives. For the dysphagic individual this isolation is highlighted every day, as family members continue their normal mealtime interactions. As swallowing specialists, SLPs attempt to help the person with dysphagia return to the family table. Initial meals, however, may consist of pureed food, if the individual is unable to swallow normal liquids. There are special powders made for this purpose, to add to liquids, in order to thicken them. But the stroke survivor may still feel isolated from the family as his meal must be different than what the others are eating.

Anarthria, or the absence of speech due to the severest form of oral weakness, leaves the stroke survivor without the ability to speak, although language function is completely preserved. This is a problem of the person who may be referred to as in a "locked in" state. He is well able to understand what is happening around him, but unable to make a sound, or perhaps even any kind of movement in response. SLPs have developed a specialty area in the treatment of the person with anarthria, providing highly technical computerized equipment, in an attempt to restore communication function. Some computerized communication systems can be operated with even a blink of an eye. But the most sophisticated computer can not replace the human ability to verbally communicate.

We will refer to two cases which illustrate the SLP's extended role in working with the communicatively impaired stroke survivor. Mr. C is a 67 year old Chinese man who experienced a stroke, following a carotid enterectomy. He presented with quite a mild dysarthria and dysphonia, and could still communicate very effectively. However, months after the stroke he remained so severely dysphagic that he required a nasogastric tube, in order to receive nutrition and hydration. He refused placement of a gastric feeding tube, as he was afraid that if he accepted such an intrusive medical treatment he would never regain the ability to eat by mouth. He was sent to us by his physician to attempt therapeutic swallowing intervention.

After we assessed Mr. C's swallowing, with the assistance of a highly specialized radiological technique known as a videofluoroscopy or X-ray study of the swallow, we felt ready to begin a treatment program. He was anxious to participate, and was most cooperative in all of the exercises that we prescribed. However, he was quite verbal in his feelings of frustration, isolation and even embarrassment at his current situation. Mr. C was a proud man who participated actively in the Chinese community, and took pride in his family. He now found himself, once dignified patriarch of the family, sitting at the end of the table with a tube taped to his nose. He felt he appeared very weak, and withdrew from family interaction. He absolutely refused to leave the house, except to attend our therapy sessions, and he referred to himself as "not a whole person."

Four months after his stroke, and about three weeks into our treatment program, Mr. C expressed great excitement. That was the day I told him he could take a small amount of food under my supervision. Imagine my surprise to find that he was not happy with the applesauce that I offered him. He wanted to know why he could not have his rice, the former mainstay of his diet. I logically explained, in my most clinical manner, that the consistency of the rice was not conducive to safe swallowing. We would have to start with applesauce and advance slowly to rice. Well, this explanation got us nowhere. Mr. C stated that he had never eaten this kind of food before, and this was not real eating. We reached a compromise when I asked him to bring a rice mixture that I knew he could manage safely. This simple switch from applesauce to a food that was an important part of his lifestyle motivated him to continue with our treatment program. Now he was able to wait until I felt it was eventually safe to recommend removal of the nasogastric tube.

By listening constructively to what our patient was telling us we were able to give this proud man back some control over his life. This allowed him to restore some sense of himself as, in his words, "a whole person." Because of this, my patient and I were able to complete his successful dysphagia rehabilitation program.

Another example is of a young woman, a mother of four children, who experienced a brainstem stroke at the age of 38. This left her so severely dysarthric that speech was a nonfunctional method of communication. Ms. S was also dysphagic, and unable to eat by mouth. She was fed by means of a nasogastric tube, which she, unfortunately, had for years, due to her medical inability to tolerate placement of a gastric tube. This stroke additionally left her without the ability to functionally use her hands. She had ataxia, or uncontrollable movements of the extremities on one side, and a dense hemiplegia on the other. She also presented with significant visual deficits and could not see beyond a shadowed image. Linguistically, Ms. S showed almost intact spelling and comprehension skills. In other words, she had the ability to formulate the language and the ideas, but was not able to motorically produce speech or write, in order to communicate. Her severe physical and communicative impairment made it necessary for her to live in an extended care facility.

Although restricted to the routine of an institution, Ms. S. was still a mother who was concerned with the lives of her four children. It was vital for her that she be able to participate in their upbringing, then being overseen by her sister. My role as an SLP involved establishing a method of communication which would allow Ms. S to participate in daily activities and communicate her needs and intentions to staff and family. She was mechanically able to quickly learn the operation of the electronic communication device I prescribed for her. However, this did not solve the multiple issues that arose from her disability. As the months progressed, Ms. S became withdrawn, and cut off contact with her family. Perhaps the strongest indication of how she viewed herself was her steadfast refusal to ever look in a mirror. She was very concerned with her severe drooling, and carried a towel with her at all times. This contributed to her difficulties with self-image.

To address these concerns and those of many other severely communicatively impaired stroke survivors, I was fortunate to have an opportunity to co-lead the Anarthria Psychotherapy Group. Working with a clinical psychologist, this unique group utilized alternative communication devices, from letter boards to computers. These were designed to facilitate communicative interaction among nonspeaking individuals. Some of the issues I watched our psychologist address for Ms. S included her continuing role as mother. That involved taking an active role in her own medical treatment, and learning to accept herself as a stroke survivor. As her clinician it was my role to help her through these issues, especially as I was the person most able to troubleshoot her communication device. It was through her continued struggle during these group treatment sessions that Ms. S began to assert herself. She even became an advocate for her communicatively impaired peers. Although she has continued to live in the extended care facility, Ms. S also resumed contact with her children, through letters she was able to create with her communication device.

The survivor of a stroke has many different problems to face, and must work with a variety of specialists on his team. The *SLP* has a unique role in that healing, and must work with the client, as a person of many parts. Experiences like those with Mr. C and Ms. S enable me to appreciate that speech treatment encompasses much more than providing the technology to allow communication. As the physicist Steven Hawking has stated, "The ability to communicate is what makes us human." The SLP is there to bridge the gap that is created when that ability is lost.

The Role of Physical Therapy in Multidisciplinary Stroke Rehabilitation

Jennifer A. Brennan

The purpose of this section is to describe the physical therapist's role in multidisciplinary stroke rehabilitation. Physical therapy intervention will be broken down into four processes including evaluation, goal setting and program planning, treatment implementation and discharge planning. It is important to state that these processes are not sequential events, but rather, they are ongoing and overlapping.

PHYSICAL THERAPY EVALUATION

Evaluation of the patient with stroke includes the assessment of:

1. *Motor Status:* The patient's ability to move various joints is tested and is often rated using the Brunnstrom stages of recovery (Flaccid, Associated Reactions, Partial Synergy, Full Synergy, Partially Isolated, Fully Isolated).
2. *Muscle Tone:* Is tested by rapidly ranging a joint and grading the resistance to PROM (hypotonic, normal, or minimally moderately or severely increased tone) or by grading DTR's (0-4).
3. *Strength:* The strength of the uninvolved and isolated extremities is measured on a scale of 0 to 5, or Zero to Normal.

Jennifer A. Brennan, MS, is Physical Therapy Supervisor of the stroke unit at the Burke Rehabilitation Hospital.

[Haworth co-indexing entry note]: "The Role of Physical Therapy in Multidisciplinary Stroke Rehabilitation." Brennan, Jennifer A. Co-published simultaneously in *Loss, Grief & Care* (The Haworth Press, Inc.) Vol. 8, No. 1/2, 1998, pp. 109-114; and: *After Stroke: Enhancing Quality of Life* (ed: Wallace Sife) The Haworth Press, Inc., 1998, pp. 109-114. Single or multiple copies of this article are available for a fee from The Haworth Document Delivery Service [1-800-342-9678, 9:00 a.m. - 5:00 p.m. (EST). E-mail address: getinfo@haworth.com].

109

4. *Sensation:* The patient's ability is evaluated to detect and locate the following stimuli: deep and light touch, sharp and dull touch, hot and cold temperature. Proprioception and kinesthesia are also tested.
5. *Balance:* Static and dynamic, sitting and standing balance are measured, using timing tests and by eliciting equilibrium and protective extension reactions (this is usually graded Poor to Normal).
6. *Range of Motion:* The physical therapist identifies limitations in the flexibility of joints. When limitations are present, goniometric measurements are recorded.
7. *Respiratory Status:* Is evaluated by determining the patient's breathing pattern, evaluating breath sounds and assessing the effectiveness of the patient's cough.
8. *Mobility:* A large part of the physical therapy evaluation consists of assessing the patient's ability to perform functional tasks. The physical therapist determines the patient's ability to perform activities such as: rolling in bed, sitting up and lying down, transferring from one surface to another, ambulating on various surfaces, negotiation of stairs and curbs and the ability to get on and off the floor. The therapist defines how much word assistance is required for each task, on a scale from total assistance to independent. In addition, the therapist evaluates the patient's safety, efficiency, endurance, vital sign changes and quality of movement when performing these tasks.

Interdisciplinary Communication

Effective rehabilitation of the patient with stroke requires close communication between interdisciplinary team members. Rather than using their evaluation findings in isolation, physical therapists consider information gathered by the physician, nursing staff, the social worker, and occupational and speech therapists. A patient's performance in physical therapy will be greatly influenced by his/her medical status, cognitive status, communication skills, perceptual skills, emotional status, level of motivation and support system.

Goal Setting and Program Planning

Once the initial evaluation is complete, the physical therapist sets short and long-term goals for the patient. These goals will determine treatment priorities and direct the plan of care. In order to maximize outcomes, it is important that goals are realistic, yet challenging. It is also important that some of the goals are directed towards the patient achieving independence. In some instances it is appropriate for the patient and his/her family to identify their own realistic goals with the guidance of the physical therapist. This empowers patients and their family members to set priorities and take some control over the course of their treatment. When the physical therapist sets the goals, it is important that the patient be made aware of these goals. Usually, there is increased compliance when the patient clearly understands the desired outcome. Finally, it is important for the interdisciplinary team to be familiar with each other's goals. This enables the team to provide the patient with more consistent care and feedback.

Projecting Outcomes

Typically, for those patients with pure motor deficits, the goal is to be independent with all mobility upon discharge. In cases where patients have motor and sensory or motor, sensory and visual deficits, the goal at the time of discharge is not independence with all mobility. Rather, the goals are to decrease the amount of assistance the patient requires, and to train family members or a caretaker to assist the patient with mobility.[1]

TREATMENT IMPLEMENTATION

Physical therapy treatment of the patient with stroke is aimed at improving his/her mobility and level of independence by attempting to reverse primary effects of stroke, teaching compensatory strategies, reversing or preventing the secondary effects of stroke, and by educating the family members who will assume the role of caretaker.

Reversing the Primary Effects of Stroke

The physical therapist attempts to improve motor control and balance and normalize tone using a variety of treatment techniques. These techniques include:

1. *Brunnstrom*, which assumes that there are normal stages of recovery after stroke (see Evaluation of Motor Status). The Brunnstrom approach uses facilitation techniques such as tonic reflexes, associated reactions, tapping, resistance, quick stretches, and voice commands to elicit muscle contractions.[2]
2. *Proprioceptive Neuromuscular Facilitation (PNF)*, which is based upon the principles of normal human development (mass movements precede individual movements, reflexive movements precede volitional movements, developments occurs cephally to caudally,

control is gained proximally prior to distally and the timing of normal movements is distal to proximal). Diagonal patterns of movement that occur frequently in common tasks are facilitated (via stretching, traction, approximation and resistance) and used to assist motor learning by increasing sensory input. These coordinated movements are practiced repeatedly to increase strength and endurance and improve timing.[3]

3. *Neuro-Developmental Treatment (NDT)/Bobath Approach.* This aims to inhibit abnormal tone and reflexes and facilitate normal movement by activating normal righting and equilibrium reactions, allowing the patient to feel normal movements and by preventing the patient from using compensatory movements.[4]

4. *Motor Relearning Program (MRP).* This is the Carr and Shepherd approach, based on the requirements for acquisition of skill or normal motor learning principles. Treatment focus is aimed at eliminating unnecessary muscle activity and providing the type of feedback and practice environments that expedite skill acquisitions.[5]

Compensatory Strategies

If the patient's deficits are profound, or there has been little to no reversal of the primary deficits, the therapist may increase the patient's function and level of independence by employing compensatory techniques. Compensations may include the use of assistive devices, such as walkers or canes, bracing such as ankle-foot orthotics or knee-ankle-foot orthotics, or instruction in alternate ways to perform once-routine tasks. For example, rather than negotiating steps with a typical step-over-step pattern, the patient may be taught to use a step-to-step pattern so that the feet come together on each step and the intact leg carries the majority of the weight.

Reversing or Preventing Secondary Deficits

Unfortunately, in addition to the primary deficits of CVA, secondary deficits such as pneumonia, contractures, deep vein thromboses, decubiti and deconditioning are common. Early physical therapy intervention is highly successful at preventing, or in some cases, reversing these deficits through ROM, chest PT, posture and mobility training.

Family Education

When it is evident that the patient will not be independent in all aspects of mobility and that a family member will be acting as a caregiver, family education becomes a treatment priority. Family members are invited to participate in therapy on a regular basis. Gradually, they are trained to be safe in assisting the patient in activities such as transfers, ambulation, stair negotiation and rising after a fall. When the patient and family member have achieved a satisfactory level of trust and comfort, and work safely together, they are given permission to practice these activities during the evenings or on weekends, without the supervision of the physical therapist. Eventually, a therapeutic pass may be recommended. The patient and family member leave the hospital for a few hours, and practice functioning in the community or in their home setting. When they return to the hospital they discuss problems that arose, so these issues can be addressed during physical therapy.

Discharge Planning

The ultimate goal of physical therapy is to discharge the patient with stroke to a safe environment where he/she can be as mobile as possible, either independently or with assistance. Patients' feelings at discharge vary. Some are very confident, and believe that discharge means they have been cured. These patients need to be cautioned about the new challenges they will face outside the rehabilitation environment. Other patients are depressed because they are not satisfied with their physical status and feel that discharge from rehabilitation is equated with the end of their recovery.

All patients need to know that recovery after stroke is a long-term process that does not end with discharge from the rehabilitation hospital. Follow-up physical therapy is usually recommended, either on an outpatient or home-care basis. This follow-up care is important to assist the patient and caregiver in their transition to the home and community. Also, patients and caregivers can be trained in home exercise programs to maintain or increase strength, endurance and range of motion. Because stroke is a long-term disability, and there are often changes in the patient's status over a long period of time, intermittent physical therapy sessions are beneficial to update patients' exercise programs or to progress patients to a new level of mobility.

NOTES

1. Reding, M.J., Potes E. Rehabilitation Outcomes Following Initial Unilateral Hemispheric Stroke. *Stroke* 1988; 19:1354-1358.
2. Brunnstrom, S. Movement Therapy in Hemiplegia. NY: Harper & Row, 1970.

3. Voss, D.E., Ionta, M.K., Myers, B.J. Proprioceptive Neuromuscular Facilitation. Philadelphia: Harper & Row, 1985.

4. Bobath, B. Adult Hemiplegia: Evaluation and Treatment. London, William Heineman Medical Books Limited, 1978, pp. 3, 58-62.

5. Carr, J.H., Shepherd, R.B. A Motor Relearning Programme for Stroke. London: Aspen Systems Corporation, 1983, pp. 3-7.

Occupational Therapy Intervention in the Rehabilitation of Stroke Patients

Eleanor Haid

This chapter concerns areas of occupational therapy intervention in the rehabilitation of stroke patients. It includes assessment, treatment goals and treatment plans for these patients. Although the areas discussed are the main focus of occupational therapy intervention in the early stages, rehabilitation requires a team effort and there are many areas that overlap. There are seven general areas of OT intervention.

1. Activities of Daily Living (ADL). At a basic level this includes eating, dressing, grooming, hygiene, bathing, functional mobility, position changes in bed, transfers to bed, toilet, tub and car, and wheelchair propulsion. It also includes functional communication, such as the ability to call for assistance in an emergency or the ability to operate the telephone.
2. Instrumental Activities of Daily Living (IADL). At an advanced level, ADL includes meal preparation, homemaking, shopping and functional activities related to home management (i.e., functional math). The care of others, educational or vocational responsibilities, hobbies and leisure time interests are also included. Leisure time interests are also addressed by the Therapeutic Recreation Department.
3. The third area that we look at is Motor Ability and Sensory Function. This includes postural reflexes, motor use of the trunk, use of

Eleanor Haid, MSEd, OTR, is Director of Occupational Therapy at Burke Rehabilitation Hospital, White Plains, NY.

[Haworth co-indexing entry note]: "Occupational Therapy Intervention in the Rehabilitation of Stroke Patients." Haid, Eleanor. Co-published simultaneously in *Loss, Grief & Care* (The Haworth Press, Inc.) Vol. 8, No. 1/2, 1998, pp. 115-122; and: *After Stroke: Enhancing Quality of Life* (ed: Wallace Sife) The Haworth Press, Inc., 1998, pp. 115-122. Single or multiple copies of this article are available for a fee from The Haworth Document Delivery Service [1-800-342-9678, 9:00 a.m. - 5:00 p.m. (EST). E-mail address: getinfo@haworth.com].

the upper extremity–particularly in relation to its use during ADL, selective movement patterns and functional use in the upper body, gross and fine motor coordination; object manipulation; and finally exercises and positioning to maintain range of motion, reduce tone, and prevent shoulder-hand syndrome and edema.

4. Visual Motor Perception.
5. Cognition.
6. Durable Medical Equipment/Positioning Equipment and Adaptive Devices. This includes prescription of wheelchairs and hospital beds, wheelchair cushions and lap boards, bathroom equipment recommendations, ADL devices such as one-handed shoe lace locks, long-handled shoe horns, and other items. Occupational Therapists also design and fabricate custom ADL devices that are not commercially available, that enable the patient to become more independent. We problem solve together with the patient, then design and make items such as one-handled insulin bottle holders, etc. Adaptations might include something as simple as putting velcro closures on clothing. Occupational therapists also fabricate custom hand splints. We sometimes provide prefabricated splints, but they generally don't fit as well.
7. The final area includes Patient Education, Family Training, and Home Programs.

POST-STROKE DEFICIT AREAS

This includes some of the typical deficit areas, or a combination of them, that are seen after a stroke. They can interfere with a patient's ability to perform ADL, independently.

MOTOR PARALYSIS

This includes weakness of the trunk, upper extremity and lower extremity on the affected side, which will interfere with ability to complete ADL. Patients with hemiparesis tend to shift all of their weight onto the unaffected side and avoid movement towards the hemiplegic side. This makes it difficult to complete lower extremity dressing. In addition, a person with hemiparesis often experiences loss of postural reflexes, loss of normal righting reactions and loss of protective reflexes. If they try to get dressed while sitting on the edge of the bed and they lean forward to put their pants leg on, they may lose their balance to the affected side. Along with weakness of the trunk muscles, they have lost the normal protective reflexes that should prevent them from falling. Once they start to fall they have difficulty in coming back to an upright position. Spasticity throughout the hemiplegic side often interferes with independence in ADL. When the extremities are tight due to spasticity, it may be troublesome to get clothing over the arm or the leg, and if the hand is closed in a tight fist, it is difficult to maintain hygiene, wash the hand and keep the skin clean.

People with painful shoulder-hand-syndrome avoid moving the arm because it hurts. They may have extreme difficulty with dressing and grooming, if it involves moving or touching a painful limb. Hemiparesis and loss of selective movement patterns of the upper extremity require the patient to use one-handed techniques for activities that are normally completed with two hands. Difficulty with fine motor coordination (FMC) in the unaffected arm may impair ability to perform ADL. FMC is commonly impaired in a stroke patient because of weakness, tremors, apraxia or difficulty with motor planning. There is a need to learn how to perform various activities with the non-dominant hand.

There are several kinds of functional problems that interfere with ADL. These include problems with sitting and standing balance, ability to change the position of the body in the bed or chair, ability to weight bear and support themselves on their affected side, ability to move the arm and the leg on the affected side, ability to ambulate, poor endurance, and poor functional use of the upper extremity due to weakness, spasticity or pain.

A secondary problem that we see is poor sitting position in the wheelchair, which puts the patient in a poor position to complete ADL. For example, the patient may be unable to reach a table for eating, unable to weight shift for dressing, or may not be in a correct position to swallow properly. Poor position may increase abnormal tone, which creates other problems in therapy, and increases the risk of skin breakdown. On the stroke unit, we spend a lot of time making sure that the person has a wheelchair that is the correct size and height, and has the proper cushions and back supports, so ADL can be effectively performed.

SENSORY DISTURBANCE

This is the next area that interferes with ADL independence. Sensation can either be impaired or absent on the affected side. Common deficits include decreased sensitivity to touch, pain, temperature, pressure, vibration or proprioception. Functionally, the kinds of problems we see in ADL may include decreased safety, e.g., the person may be unaware of balance loss or the person may touch a hot stove with the affected upper extremity and may not be aware of the burn. With proprioceptive deficits, there is poor awareness of the location of body parts. Some examples of this are poor placement of the foot during ambulation (resulting in balance problems), difficulty pushing the arm through the sleeve of clothing, especially when the vision is occluded, or poor positioning of the upper extremity during position changes (which could result in injury). Frequently the patient rolls toward the unaffected side. All team members reinforce an awareness in the patient that the involved extremity must be positioned first to decrease the risk of painful shoulder-hand syndrome.

PERCEPTUAL DYSFUNCTION

This is the next area that may interfere with ADL independence. The most common deficits occur in the areas of visual perception, body awareness and motor planning. Problems with visual spatial awareness or the ability to detect subtle or gross differences in position, direction, angle and rotations may occur. The person may have difficulty orienting his body in space, and in perceiving the position of objects in relation to himself. Functionally, the types of problems in ADL include difficulty estimating object size or distance, difficulty in orienting an object (putting on a shirt, for example). He may also have difficulty following a route through the hospital, and trouble positioning objects during construction tasks. Difficulty in orienting objects for construction may be observed in activities such as building a sandwich or wrapping a package.

The next area under perceptual dysfunction is body awareness. A person may have difficulty in integrating the relationship of the body parts to the whole body. There may be problems with orientation of the body in space, such as difficulty in sitting upright, difficulty with midline orientation, problems with right/left discrimination, unilateral inattention or the lack of use of one side of the body, even in the absence of sensory or motor problems. One may observe difficulty with bilateral integration and in sequencing the steps of the task. Functionally, other problems that can be seen include difficulty following verbal or written directions, difficulty using both upper extremities in a coordinated fashion, difficulty with mobility activities (such as propelling the wheelchair, making turns in the wheelchair, and pulling up to a table), difficulty maintaining posture during dynamic tasks such as dressing, and failure to attend to one side of the body. Examples of unilateral inattention include shaving one side of the face and not the other, or eating from the one side of the plate but not from the other. Examples of difficulty performing the steps of an activity may be seen during preparation to do a stand-pivot transfer from the wheelchair to the bed. Steps taught include, pulling up next to the bed, locking the brakes, removing legs from the leg rest, lifting the foot plates up, swinging the leg rests away, and pulling forward in the chair. A person may have difficulty sequencing those steps and executing them in the correct order. At a higher level, a person might have difficulty driving a car or following a sequence of directions.

The next area under perceptual dysfunction is motor planning. Problems may occur with either the production of movement or the conceptualization of how to do the task or use an object. Functionally, problems may occur with either the timing or the execution of the movement, and are noticed especially during activities that require fine motor control. Gross motor control may also be affected. We may observe poor ability to learn new motor movements—for example, difficulty in learning one handed techniques to compensate for hemiplegia. Another motor planning problem is preservation or repetition of a motor pattern. A person may get stuck and be unable to go on to the next step of the activity. Perseveration is very obvious when it is observed on paper, when a patient attempts to write. But perseveration can be manifested much more subtly. Patients may get stuck on an activity that they were working on in their previous program, and may want to continue with that activity or conversation. They may be unable to break out of that pattern to move on to the next thing.

VISUAL DISTURBANCES

These may be considered as a separate category. Vision is integrated with all of the other areas. When a person has visual deficits, usually there are severe problems with ADL. Homonymous hemianopsia is an inability to detect stimuli in either the right or left half of both visual fields. A person with hemianopsia in whom cognition and perception are intact can learn to compensate for the hemianopsia with training. Unilateral visual inattention or inattention to stimuli in one visual field is a much more difficult problem. Remediation techniques are often not as successful, and deficits in ADL may occur. Other visual problems that occur are motor impersistence (decreased ability to maintain visual fixation on an object or work), decreased visual search into the affected visual field, and decreased scanning. Functionally, there will be problems in self-care. The person may miss objects on one side of the plate, or objects that are one side of their body, during grooming. When reading they may miss words or letters on half or part of the page. They may have difficulty scanning from left to right or scanning effectively from line to line, and they may have trouble fixating on words. During functional math activities, we see the same types of problems and the same types of errors with check book calculations and reading financial statements. Visual deficits such as these may also prevent return to driving.

COGNITIVE AND PERSONALITY CHANGES

Two other problems that may impact on ADL are changes in cognition and personality. The most common difficulties we see are distractibility, decreased attention, poor memory (especially for new learning), lack of insight, rigidity and lack of initiation. Some patients may not initiate self-care or other activities unless prodded by the staff. Some patients utilize poor judgement and may be completely unaware that they are in an unsafe situation. They may be impulsive, have low frustration tolerance, emotional lability, depression, denial and poor self esteem. Any of these changes may interfere with independence in ADL.

AUDITORY LANGUAGE DEFICITS

Auditory or receptive/expressive language deficits can interfere with independence in ADL. When a person has difficulty hearing, he will have difficulty following verbal directions. If there is a misperception of words, it can lead to incorrect performance. In either case, the patient may have difficulty sustaining attention to ADL tasks that require verbal instructions. Here, the task requires a much greater effort, and can cause fatigue. The patient may become frustrated because he does not understand the types of cues the therapist has given him.

Problems with any one of these areas can contribute to decreased independence in ADL. The impact of psychosocial, motor, sensory, cognitive and perceptual changes must be analyzed to determine which components are most interfering with a positive outcome. After the deficits that most interfere with function are carefully defined, a comprehensive treatment plan can be developed. For example, three different patients are unable to dress themselves. One patient can't accomplish this because his trunk and extremities are weak and he can't balance or position his body to don clothing. Treatment would involve strengthening the trunk and extremity muscles, teaching correct position change techniques, and improving balance, before teaching one-handed techniques. This person may very well become independent, even with severe motor problems. A second patient may have poor awareness of the left side of his body, and intact function in the left upper extremity and trunk. Although intact motorically he only dresses the right side of his body, and totally ignores the left. Treatment before initiating an ADL training program might consist of gross motor bilateral activities (to increase awareness of the left side of the body) and visual scanning activities. A third person may have difficulty with sequencing or spatial awareness, and the approach would be totally different. Training techniques may include verbal rehearsal, visual cues or diagrams of the sequence of steps used. Adaptive techniques, such as teaching the person to locate the landmarks on the shirt, can make spatial orientation easier. For example, the tag can be used to orient the shirt properly, before one starts dressing. A careful analysis of interfering factors is required.

In some rehab programs a great emphasis is placed on treatment of motor dysfunction because the patient and family tend to focus on it. But there are many less-visible problems that have a much greater impact on patient performance in ADL, than motor status alone. Comprehensive occupational therapy and team evaluation are necessary. The evaluation findings of all team members are shared. The team can then decide which goals can be realistically achieved during the rehab phase. This information must be communicated clearly to the family and to the patients, so everyone has realistic expectations of the outcome of the program. Very few severely disabled patients return home after rehab totally independent in ADL. From an OT perspective, continued assistance is usually maintained for safety reasons. The patients need to rely very heavily on their family or caregivers, in the early months after rehab. The family must be knowledgeable about the patient's status, and understand the specific reasons why that person requires assistance. This helps to prepare the family for the amount of effort that is necessary to maintain the patient at home, helps them to develop realistic expectations of the patient's abilities, and helps them to use the correct strategies to maximize the patient's performance. It allows them to help the patient to make progress at home after discharge and also helps them to cope with the inevitable stress that results from the role changes, the frustration, the physical and emotional drain on them that will occur in the next few months after the patient returns home.

At Burke we have several ways of facilitating this process with the patient's family, prior to discharge. This first is a day of observation in which the family observes the patient in all of the therapy programs. The purpose is to familiarize the family with the patient's abilities and needs. In OT, the family has an opportunity to practice activities such as transfers, in order to feel how much physical assistance is required. During this visit, we tentatively review durable medical equipment (DME) recommendations. This allows the family to begin planning for the transition to home.

The second technique is a focused training session, used for additional instruction in any area, as often as necessary. Prior to the issuance of a day pass, the family will come in for intensive training in toileting and car transfers, until they feel comfortable with assisting the patient. Some sessions are used to review the home exercise program, especially upper extremity exercises. DME problem solving and training might also be reviewed. The day pass is a very important tool because it provides the patient and family an opportunity to try these techniques in their home environment. When they come back, they give us a lot of feedback on performance and we can adjust our treatment program accordingly.

The third technique is the family conference, which is a meeting between the family and all the team members. Team members summarize the patient's status, the amount of physical assistance required, the number of hours and type of care that will be required upon return to the community. They then outline goals, and allow the family to give input on goals. They discuss anticipated length of stay so the family can start planning for discharge. We also review home equipment recommendations and the cost of that equipment, as it can be quite expensive. We recommend follow-up therapy and services, if necessary.

A fourth technique is to either do a home evaluation or ask the family to fill out a questionnaire and take home measurements to determine accessibility and DME needs. The last area of family preparation is stroke education. To help cope with stroke and get back into the mainstream of life, there are daytime classes for the patients on various topics, and family training sessions, given in the evenings.

Therapeutic Recreation
and the Rehabilitation of the Stroke Patient

Joanne Auerbach
Allan Benezra

OVERVIEW

Therapeutic recreation can play an important role in the rehabilitation of the person who has had a stroke. Early and continued intervention by the therapeutic recreation specialist can be especially effective in addressing psychosocial issues encountered by the patient. Fear, anger, frustration, depression, hopelessness, loss of independence, altered body image, diminished abilities, damaged self-image, uncertainty about the future, and a diminished sense of control are issues as real as more easily measured physical deficits. If not addressed, these less tangible results of stroke can present serious barriers to improvement in overall function. Through a carefully planned process of individual and/or group interventions, the recreation therapist helps the patient (and the patient's family) regain a sense of wholeness and hope, and consequently, improved function and quality of life.

The first step in this process is an initial assessment to determine the patient's current status. By definition, the purpose of therapeutic recreation is to improve/maintain physical, cognitive, social and/or emotional

Joanne Auerbach, MA CTRS, is a certified recreational therapist, and Director of Recreational Therapy at Burke Rehabilitation Hospital. Allan Benezra, MS, CTRS, is a certified recreational therapist and is currently serving as therapeutic Recreational Supervisor at Burke Rehabilitation Hospital, White Plains, NY.

[Haworth co-indexing entry note]: "Therapeutic Recreation and the Rehabilitation of the Stroke Patient." Auerbach, Joanne, and Allan Benezra. Co-published simultaneously in *Loss, Grief & Care* (The Haworth Press, Inc.) Vol. 8, No. 1/2, 1998, pp. 123-128; and: *After Stroke: Enhancing Quality of Life* (ed: Wallace Sife) The Haworth Press, Inc., 1998, pp. 123-128. Single or multiple copies of this article are available for a fee from The Haworth Document Delivery Service [1-800-342-9678, 9:00 a.m. - 5:00 p.m. (EST). E-mail address: getinfo@haworth.com].

123

functioning. Consequently, the recreation therapy assessment gathers information in these areas, and includes information on the patient's previous leisure lifestyle. Long term goals and short term objectives are established, and a treatment plan is developed. In addition to individual therapy sessions, the patient may be referred to any number of recreation therapy groups (such as cognitive stimulation, leisure education, etc.). The therapist involves family members in the assessment process and in the development of the treatment plan, especially in cases where the patient's ability to comprehend and process information is limited.

Interventions

Some common problems experienced by the stroke patient are discussed below, along with a brief overview of some treatment interventions employed by a recreation therapist.

Cognitive Deficits

Recreational activities conducted in small groups or on a one-to-one basis can be used to address cognitive deficits following a stroke. Age-appropriate, simplified activities which are interesting to the patient are used by the recreation therapist to address areas such as disorientation, decreased alertness, shortened attention span, and memory deficits. Orientation to time, for example, may be reinforced through seasonal/holiday activities, current events discussions, and through observation and experience of the weather and outdoor environment. Simple craft projects can provide practice in sequencing, following directions, and processing new information. Group games are used to increase the patient's awareness of others who are participating, and to stimulate thought processes. Reminiscence activities using verbal, visual, and/or musical stimuli enable patients to draw on distant memory of younger days, family life, achievements, and fun times. The recreational therapist helps the patient make then-now connections and reinforces the patient's sense of self. Repetition and reinforcement aid with short term and recent memory, as activities are recalled from the beginning of a session to the end, and from one session to another.

Depression and Isolation

The grieving process for what has been lost often results in feelings of depression, and the patient may become isolated and withdrawn. The recreational therapist attempts to help the patient (and family) through these feelings to a more hopeful and positive outlook, both in a formal way during therapy sessions, and informally in the patient's free time. Drawing on the patient's previous leisure interests, the therapist aims to gradually re-engage the patient in enjoyable and uplifting experiences. While acknowledging the patient's feelings of loss as valid, the therapist uses recreational activities to allow the patient and family opportunities to experience that life still has promise for continued fun and laughter. Social and cultural programs, music, and humor can be effective tools to this end. Diversional activities, by their nature, are beneficial to both the patient and the patient's family.

Stress

Frustration, uncertainty about the future, and anger may lead to high levels of stress. Not only are these feelings distressing to the patient, they often hinder the effectiveness of other treatment modalities. The recreation therapist addresses the issue of stress in a number of ways. Engaging the patient in leisure activities he or she previously enjoyed can be effective in diverting attention away from stressful thoughts. Family members, too, are encouraged to engage in recreational outlets, both with the patient and separately. This process allows the patient and family to feel less fragmented, and better able to cope. Listening to music, use of relaxation tapes, and exposure to peaceful natural surroundings can help reduce tension. Creative pursuits such as painting, collages, or writing can also be effective outlets for stress.

Loss of Confidence

In the face of the limitations caused by stroke, the patient may feel discouraged, and have lowered self-confidence. The recreational therapist addresses this issue, in part, by engaging the patient in experiences at which he or she can be successful. Although these successes may be small in the beginning, the therapist will gradually increase the perceived difficulty so that feelings of mastery and self-confidence build. Since leisure experiences are usually self-motivating, the patient becomes invested in the process.

The therapist also helps the patient overcome problems which prevent participation in previously enjoyed recreational activities. Some solutions are relatively simple and concrete. An individual may perceive, for example, that he or she can no longer play cards because hemiplegia has made holding and shuffling awkward or impossible. The therapist will introduce a card holder and automatic shuffler, instruct the patient on their use, and practice some card games that the patient enjoys. Solutions lead to success, which in turn leads to increased confidence.

Other interventions are less tangible. Reminiscing activities, such as those mentioned above, also influence perceived competence.

Community re-entry is an especially significant area about which patients may feel uneasy. They may wonder if they will be stared at, if physical barriers will prevent participation, if they have the necessary endurance, and how they will handle their bathroom needs. Under the supervision of the recreation therapist, a group outing to a movie, concert, play, shopping mall, or baseball game is often a confidence builder. Such experiences afford an opportunity to practice skills learned in other therapies, as well. An accessibility checklist given to the patient and family helps to ensure successful and satisfying experiences in the community after discharge from the hospital.

MEANINGFUL USE OF DISCRETIONARY TIME

Deterioration in leisure activities was the foremost problem following stroke as reported by 80% of one study population reported in *Stroke* (Niemi et al., 1988). It follows, then, that a significant role of the recreational therapist is to address the issue of barriers to participation in satisfying leisure activities. These barriers may include the following:

1. *The Patient's Lack of Awareness of His/Her Own Leisure Lifestyle.* Many persons (whether disabled or not) are unable to articulate their own leisure interests, motivations and satisfactions. Some strongly work-oriented individuals may actually have a negative attitude with regard to the concept of leisure, viewing it as insignificant or trivial. These individuals may nonetheless find themselves with a substantial amount of discretionary time following a stroke or other disabling condition. Through numerous assessments and leisure education tools (both verbal and non-verbal) the recreational therapist can assist the patient in identifying those pursuits which he or she previously enjoyed. The therapist can also help the patient and the family understand how leisure pursuits have filled a variety of needs, such as intellectual stimulation, the desire to feel productive and useful, social interaction, relaxation, artistic expression, physical and spiritual well-being, exhilaration, peacefulness, and competence, just to name a few. Continued participation in recreational activities following stroke, both in the hospital and after discharge, can increase overall life satisfaction by continuing to fulfill needs.

2. *Limited Leisure Repertoire.* Some patients have, in fact, only a few leisure interests. This situation is problematic if the patient is unable to continue with some of these (thus having an even smaller repertoire to choose from) and/or if the patient has significantly more discretionary time (thus having more hours to fill). Based on the patient's values, motivations, and previous sources of fulfillment, the therapist can introduce new activities which the patient will find satisfying. Sometimes leisure interests which have been long dormant are rekindled and enjoyed.

3. *Perceived Inability to Continue Previous Leisure Interests.* Whether the activity which the patient thinks is "over" is relatively simple or quite complex, the recreational therapist is a source of information, advice, and resource materials. For the person who liked to read, but can no longer do so because of perceptual difficulties or other impairment following stroke, talking books can be a viable alternative. The therapist can assist the patient in making arrangements for having this free service at home. The patient who had enjoyed traveling may assume that this pursuit now presents nearly insurmountable difficulties. The information that the recreational therapist can provide (on general planning tips for persons with disabilities, transportation considerations, organizations which specialize in assisting "challenged" travelers, etc.) can literally open a world of possibilities for the stroke patient and his or her family. These are only a few examples of the many ways that the recreational therapist assists the patient to identify and overcome barriers to participation in satisfying leisure activities.

CONCLUSION

Stroke is a devastating experience with negative effects on physical, cognitive, social, and emotional functioning. All of these areas are important to the patient's well-being, and all are interdependent. As part of the rehabilitation team, the recreational therapist addresses these issues through a variety of treatment interventions, only a few of which could be mentioned here. From admission to discharge and beyond, the recreational therapist works together with all members of the healthcare team to improve function and quality of life, so the patient and family together can look ahead with increased hope and optimism.

REFERENCES

Baines, S., Saxby, R, & Ehlert, K. (1987, August). Reality Orientation and Reminiscence Therapy: A Controlled Cross-Over Study of Elderly Confused People. *British Journal of Psychiatry,* 151, 222-231.

Berk, L. et al. (1988). Humor Associated Laughter Decreases Cortisol and Increases Spontaneous Lymphocyte Blastogenesis. *Clinical Research*, 36, 435.

Caplan, B., ed. (1987). *Rehabilitation Psychology Desk Reference.* Rockville, MD: Aspen.

Citrin, R. & Dixon, D. (1977). Reality Orientation: A Milieu Therapy Used in an Institution for the Aged. *Gerontologist,* 17, 39-43.

Cousins, N. (1980). *Anatomy of an Illness.* Boston: G. K. Hall.

Cousins, N. (1989). *Head First: The Biology of Hope.* New York: Dutton.

Coyle, C. P., & Kinney, W. B., Riley, B., & Shank, J., eds. (1991). *Benefits of Therapeutic Recreation: A Consensus View.* Ravendale, WA: Idyll Arbor, Inc.

Fry, W., Jr., M.D. & Salameh, W., eds. (1987). *Handbook of Humor and Psychotherapy: Advances in the Clinical Use of Humor.* Sarasota, Florida: Professional Resources Exchange.

Giordano, D. & Everly, G. (1979). *Controlling Stress and Tension: A Holistic Approach.* Englewood Cliffs, NJ: Prentice-Hall.

Godbey, G. (1990). *Leisure in your life: An exploration.* State College, PA: Venture.

Harrell, M., Parente, F., Bellingrath, E., & Liscia, K. (1992). *Cognitive Rehabilitation of Memory: A Practical Guide.* Gathersburg, MD: Aspen.

Haun, P. (1966). *Recreation: A Medical Viewpoint.* New York: Teachers College Press.

Heywood, L. A. (1978). Perceived Recreation Experience and the Relief of Tension. *Journal of Leisure Research,* 10, 86-97.

Mandrell, A. R., & Keller, S. M. (1986). Stress Management in Rehabilitation. *Archives of Physical Medicine and Rehabilitation,* 67, 375-379.

Nahemow, L., McCluckey-Fawcett, K., & McGhee, P., eds. (1986). *Humor and Aging.* San Diego, CA: Academic Press, Inc.

Niemi, M. L., Laaksonen, R., Kotila, M., & Wattimo, O. (1988). Quality of Life Four Years After Stroke. *Stroke,* 19(9), 1101-1107.

Reigler, J. (1980). Comparison of a Reality Orientation Program for Geriatric Patients With and Without Music. *Journal of Music Therapy,* 17, 26-33.

Schafer, D., Berghorn, R, Holmes, D., & Quadagno, J. (1986). The Effects of Reminiscing on the Perceived Control and Social Relations of Institutionalized Elderly. *Activities, Adaptation & Aging,* 8, 95-110.

Shank, J. W., Coyle, C. R, & Kinney, W. B. (1991a, September). A Comparison of the Effects of Clinical versus Diversional Therapeutic Recreation Involvement on Rehabilitation Outcomes. Paper presented at Benefits of Therapeutic Recreation in Rehabilitation Conference, Lafayette Hill, PA.

Siegel, B., M.D. (1986). *Love, Medicine and Miracles: Lessons Learned About Self-Healing From a Surgeon's Experience With Exceptional Patients.* New York: Harper & Row.

Ulrich, R. S., Dimberg, V., & Driver, B. L. (1990). Psycho-Physiological Indicators of Leisure Consequences. *Journal of Leisure Research,* 22(2), 154-166.

Weiss, C. R. (1989). T.R. and Reminiscing: The Pursuit of Elusive Memory and the Art of Remembering. *Therapeutic Recreation Journal,* 23(3), 7-18.

The Nature of Suffering
and the Goals of Medicine

Eric J. Cassell

The obligation of physicians to relieve human suffering stretches back into antiquity. Despite this fact, little attention is explicitly given to the problem of suffering in medical education, research, or practice. I will begin by focusing on a modern paradox: Even in the best settings and with the best physicians, it is not uncommon for suffering to occur not only during the course of a disease but also as a result of its treatment. To understand this paradox and its resolution requires an understanding of what suffering is and how it relates to medical care.

Consider this case: A 35-year-old sculptor with metastatic disease of the breast was treated by competent physicians employing advanced knowledge and technology, and acting out of kindness and true concern. At every stage, the treatment as well as the disease was a source of suffering to her. She was uncertain and frightened about her future, but she could get little information from her physicians, and what she was told was not always the truth. She had been unaware, for example, that the irradiated breast would be so disfigured. After an oophorectomy and a regimen of medications, she became hirsute, obese, and devoid of libido. With tumor in the supraclavicular fossa, she lost strength in the hand that she had used in sculpturing, and she became profoundly depressed. She had a pathologic fracture of the femur, and treatment was delayed while her physicians openly disagreed about pinning her hip.

Eric J. Cassell, MD, is Clinical Professor of Medical Ethics at Cornell University Medical College in New York City.

Reprinted by permission of *The New England Journal of Medicine*, Vol. 306, No. 11, March 18, 1982, 639-645.

[Haworth co-indexing entry note]: "The Nature of Suffering and the Goals of Medicine." Cassell, Eric J. Co-published simultaneously in *Loss, Grief & Care* (The Haworth Press, Inc.) Vol. 8, No. 1/2, 1998, pp. 129-142; and: *After Stroke: Enhancing Quality of Life* (ed: Wallace Sife) The Haworth Press, Inc., 1998, pp. 129-142.

Each time her disease responded to therapy and her hope was rekindled, a new manifestation would appear. Thus, when a new course of chemotherapy was started, she was torn between a desire to live and the fear that allowing hope to emerge again would merely expose her to misery if the treatment failed. The nausea and vomiting from the chemotherapy were distressing, but no more so than the anticipation of hair loss. She feared the future. Each tomorrow was seen as heralding increased sickness, pain, or disability, never as the beginning of better times. She felt isolated because she was no longer like other people and could not do what other people did. She feared that her friends would stop visiting her. She was sure that she would die.

This young woman had severe pain and other physical symptoms that caused her suffering. But she also suffered from some threats that were social, and from others that were personal and private. She suffered from the effects of the disease and its treatment on her appearance and abilities. She also suffered unremittingly from her perception of the future.

What can this case tell us about the ends of medicine and the relief of suffering? Three facts stand out: The first is that this woman's suffering was not confined to her physical symptoms. The second is that she suffered not only from her disease but also from its treatment. The third is that one could not anticipate what she would describe as a source of suffering; like other patients, she had to be asked. Some features of her condition she would call painful, upsetting, uncomfortable, and distressing, but not a source of suffering. In these characteristics her case was ordinary.

In discussing the matter of suffering with lay persons, I learned that they were shocked to discover that the problem of suffering was not directly addressed in medical education. My colleagues of a contemplative nature were surprised at how little they knew of the problem and how little thought they had given it, whereas medical students tended to be unsure of the relevance of the issue to their work.

The relief of suffering, it would appear, is considered one of the primary ends of medicine by patients and lay persons, but not by the medical profession. As in the care of the dying, patients and their friends and families do not make a distinction between physical and nonphysical sources of suffering in the same way that doctors do.[1]

A search of the medical and social-science literature did not help me in understanding what suffering is; the word "suffering" was most often coupled with the word "pain," as in "pain and suffering." (The data bases used were *Psychological Abstracts*, the *Citation Index*, and the *Index Medicus*.)

This phenomenon reflects a historically constrained and currently inadequate view of the ends of medicine. Medicine's traditional concern primarily for the body and for physical disease is well known, as are the widespread effects of the mind-body dichotomy on medical theory and practice. I believe that this dichotomy itself is a source of the paradoxical situation in which doctors cause suffering in their care of the sick. Today, as ideas about the separation of mind and body are called into question, physicians are concerning themselves with new aspects of the human condition. The profession of medicine is being pushed and pulled into new areas, both by its technology and by the demands of its patients. Attempting to understand what suffering is and how physicians might truly be devoted to its relief will require that medicine and its critics overcome the dichotomy between mind and body, and the associated dichotomies between subjective and objective, and between person and object.

In the remainder of this paper I am going to make three points. The first is that suffering is experienced by persons. In the separation between mind and body, the concept of the person, or personhood, has been associated with that of mind, spirit, and the subjective. However, as I will show, a person is not merely mind, merely spiritual, or only subjectively knowable. Personhood has many facets, and it is ignorance of them that actively contributes to patients' suffering. The understanding of the place of the person in human illness requires a rejection of the historical dualism of mind and body.

The second point derives from my interpretation of clinical observations: Suffering occurs when an impending destruction of the person is perceived; it continues until the threat of disintegration has passed or until the integrity of the person can be restored in some other manner. It follows, then, that although suffering often occurs in the presence of acute pain, shortness of breath, or other bodily symptoms, suffering extends beyond the physical. Most generally, suffering can be defined as the state of severe distress associated with events that threaten the intactness of the person.

The third point is that suffering can occur in relation to any aspect of the person, whether it is in the realm of social roles, group identification, the relation with self, body, or family, or the relation with a transpersonal, transcendent source of meaning. Below is a simplified description or "topology" of the constituents of personhood.

"PERSON" IS NOT "MIND"

The split between mind and body that has so deeply influenced our approach to medical care was proposed by Descartes to resolve certain philosophical issues. Moreover, Cartesian dualism made it possible for science to escape the control of the church by assigning the noncorporeal, spiritual realm to the church, leaving the physical world as the domain of science. In that religious age, "person," synonymous with "mind," was necessarily off limits to science.

Changes in the meaning of concepts like that of personhood occur with changes in society, while the word for the concept remains the same. This fact tends to obscure the depth of the transformations that have occurred between the 17th century and today. People simply are "persons" in this time, as in past times, and they have difficulty imagining that the term described something quite different in an earlier period when the concept was more constrained.

If the mind-body dichotomy results in assigning the body to medicine, and the person is not in that category, then the only remaining place for the person is in the category of mind. Where the mind is problematic (not identifiable in objective terms), its very reality diminishes for science, and so, too, does that of the person. Therefore, so long as the mind-body dichotomy is accepted, suffering is either subjective and thus not truly "real"–not within medicine's domain–or identified exclusively with bodily pain. Not only is such an identification misleading and distorting, for it depersonalizes the sick patient, but it is itself a source of suffering. It is not possible to treat sickness as something that happens solely to the body without thereby risking damage to the person. An anachronistic division of the human condition into what is medical (having to do with the body) and what is nonmedical (the remainder) has given medicine too narrow a notion of its calling. Because of this division, physicians may, in concentrating on the cure of bodily disease, do things that cause the patient as a person to suffer.

AN IMPENDING DESTRUCTION OF PERSON

Suffering is ultimately a personal matter. Patients sometimes report suffering when one does not expect it, or do not report suffering when one does expect it. Furthermore, a person can suffer enormously at the distress of another, especially a loved one.

In some theologies, suffering has been seen as bringing one closer to God. This "function" of suffering is at once its glorification and its relief. If, through great pain or deprivation, someone is brought closer to a cherished goal, that person may have no sense of having suffered but may instead feel enormous triumph. To an observer, however, only the deprivation may be apparent. This cautionary note is important because people are often said to have suffered greatly, in a religious context, when they are known only to have been injured, tortured, or in pain, not to have suffered.

Although pain and suffering are closely identified in the medical literature, they are phenomenologically distinct.[2] The difficulty of understanding pain and the problems of physicians in providing adequate relief of physical pain are well known.[3-5]

The greater the pain, the more it is believed to cause suffering. However, some pain, like that of childbirth, can be extremely severe and yet considered rewarding. The perceived meaning of pain influences the amount of medication that will be required to control it. For example, a patient reported that when she believed the pain in her leg was sciatica, she could control it with small doses of codeine, but when she discovered that it was due to the spread of malignant disease, much greater amounts of medication were required for relief. Patients can writhe in pain from kidney stones and by their own admission not be suffering, because they "know what it is"; they may also report considerable suffering from apparently minor discomfort when they do not know its source. Suffering in close relation to the intensity of pain is reported when the pain is virtually overwhelming, such as that associated with a dissecting aortic aneurysm. Suffering is also reported when the patient does not believe that the pain can be controlled. The suffering of patients with terminal cancer can often be relieved by demonstrating that their pain truly can be controlled; they will then often tolerate the same pain without any medication, preferring the pain to the side effects of their analgesics. Another type of pain that can be a source of suffering is pain that is not overwhelming but continues for a very long time.

In summary, people in pain frequently report suffering from the pain when they feel out of control, when the pain is overwhelming, when the source of the pain is unknown, when the meaning of the pain is dire, or when the pain is chronic.

In all these situations, persons perceive pain as a threat to their continued existence—not merely to their lives, but to their integrity as persons. That this is the relation of pain to suffering is strongly suggested by the fact that suffering can be relieved, in the presence of continued pain, by making the source of the pain known, changing its meaning, and demonstrating that it can be controlled, and that an end is in sight.

It follows, then, that suffering has a temporal element. In order for a situation to be a source of suffering, it must influence the person's perception of future events. ("If the pain continues like this, I *will be* overwhelmed"; "If the pain comes from cancer, I *will* die"; "If the pain cannot be controlled, I *will not* be able to take it.") At the moment when the patient is saying, "If the pain continues like this, I *will be* overwhelmed," he or she is not overwhelmed. Fear itself always involves the future. In the case with which I opened this paper, the patient could not give up her fears of her sense of future, despite the agony they caused her. As suffering is discussed in the other dimensions of personhood, note how it would not exist if the future were not a major concern.

Two other aspects of the relation between pain and suffering should be mentioned. Suffering can occur when physicians do not validate the patient's pain. In the absence of disease, physicians may suggest that the pain is "psychological" (in the sense of not being real) or that the patient is "faking." Similarly, patients with chronic pain may believe after a time that they can no longer talk to others about their distress. In the former case the person is caused to distrust his or her perceptions of reality, and in both instances social isolation adds to the person's suffering.

Another aspect essential to an understanding of the suffering of sick persons is the relation of meaning to the way in which illness is experienced. The word "meaning" is used here in two senses. In the first, to mean is to signify, to imply. Pain in the chest may imply heart disease. We also say that we know what something means when we know how important it is. The importance of things is always personal and individual, even though meaning in this sense may be shared by others or by society as a whole. What something signifies and how important it is relative to the whole array of a person's concerns, contribute to its personal meaning. "Belief" is another word for that aspect of meaning concerned with implications, and "value" concerns the degree of importance to a particular person.

The personal meaning of things does not consist exclusively of values and beliefs that are held intellectually; it includes other dimensions. For the same word, a person may simultaneously have a cognitive meaning, an affective or emotional meaning, a bodily meaning, and a transcendent or spiritual meaning. And there may be contradictions in the different levels of meaning. The nuances of personal meaning are complex, and when I speak of personal meanings I am implying this complexity in all its depth— known and unknown. Personal meaning is a fundamental dimension of personhood, and there can be no understanding of human illness or suffering without taking it into account.

A SIMPLIFIED DESCRIPTION OF THE PERSON

A simple topology of a person may be useful in understanding the relation between suffering and the goals of medicine. The features discussed below point the way to further study and to the possibility of specific action by individual physicians.

Persons have personality and character. Personality traits appear within the first few weeks of life and are remarkably durable over time. Some personalities handle some illnesses better than others. Individual persons vary in character as well. During the heyday of psychoanalysis in the 1950s, all behavior was attributed to unconscious determinants: No one was bad or good; they were merely sick or well. Fortunately, that simplistic view of human character is now out of favor. Some people do in fact have stronger characters and bear adversity better. Some are good and kind under the stress of terminal illness, whereas others become mean and offensive when even mildly ill.

A person has a past. The experiences gathered during one's life are a part of today as well as yesterday. Memory exists in the nostrils and the hands, not only in the mind. A fragrance drifts by, and a memory is evoked. My feet have not forgotten how to roller-skate, and my hands remember skills that I was hardly aware I had learned. When these past experiences involve sickness and medical care, they can influence present illness and medical care. They stimulate fear, confidence, physical symptoms, and anguish. It damages people to rob them of their past and deny their memories, or to mock their fears and worries. A person without a past is incomplete.

Life experiences–previous illness, experiences with doctors, hospitals, and medications, deformities and disabilities, pleasures and successes, miseries and failures–all form the nexus for illness. The personal meaning of the disease and its treatment arises from the past as well as the present. If cancer occurs in a patient with self-confidence from past achievements, it may give rise to optimism and a resurgence of strength. Even if it is fatal, the disease may not produce the destruction of the person but, rather, reaffirm his or her indomitability. The outcome would be different in a person for whom life had been a series of failures.

The intensity of ties to the family cannot be overemphasized; people frequently behave as though they were physical extensions of their parents. Events that might cause suffering in others may be borne without complaint by someone who believes that the disease is part of his or her family identity, and hence inevitable. Even diseases for which no heritable basis is known may be borne easily by a person because others in the family have been similarly afflicted. Just as the person's past experiences give meaning to present events, so do the past experiences of his or her family. Those meanings are part of the person.

A person has a cultural background. Just as a person is part of a culture and a society, these elements are part of the person. Culture defines what is meant by masculinity or femininity, what attire is acceptable, attitudes toward the dying and sick, mating behavior, the height of chairs and steps, degrees of tolerance for odors and excreta, and how the aged and the disabled are treated. Cultural definitions have an enormous impact on the sick and can be a source of untold suffering. They influence the behavior of others toward the sick person and that of the sick toward themselves. Cultural norms and social rules regulate whether someone can be among others or will be isolated, whether the sick will be considered foul or acceptable, and whether they are to be pitied or censured.

Returning to the sculptor described earlier, we know why that young woman suffered. She was housebound and bedbound, her face was changed by steroids, she was masculinized by her treatment, one breast was scarred, and she had almost no hair. The degree of importance attached to these losses—that aspect of their personal meaning—is determined to a great degree by cultural priorities.

With this in mind, we can also realize how much someone devoid of physical pain, even devoid of "symptoms" may suffer. People suffer from what they have lost of themselves in relation to the world of objects, events, and relationships. We realize, too, that although medical care can reduce the impact of sickness, inattentive care can increase the disruption caused by illness.

A person has roles. I am a husband, a father, a physician, a teacher, a brother, an orphaned son, and an uncle. People are their roles, and each role has rules. Together, the rules that guide the performance of roles make up a complex set of entitlements and limitations of responsibility and privilege. By middle age, the roles may be so firmly set that disease can lead to the virtual destruction of a person by making the performance of his or her roles impossible. Whether the patient is a doctor who cannot doctor or a mother who cannot mother, he or she is diminished by the loss of function.

No person exists without others; there is no consciousness without a consciousness of others, no speaker without a hearer, and no act, object, or thought that does not somehow encompass others.[6] All behavior is or will be involved with others, even if only in memory or reverie. Take away others, remove sight or hearing, and the person is diminished. Everyone dreads becoming blind or deaf but these are only the most obvious injuries to human interaction. There are many ways in which human beings can be cut off from others, and then suffer the loss.

It is in relationships with others that the full range of human emotions finds expression. It is this dimension of the person that may be injured when illness disrupts the ability to express emotion. Furthermore, the extent and nature of a sick person's relationships influence the degree of suffering from a disease. There is a vast difference between going home to an empty apartment and going home to a network of friends and family, after hospitalization. Illness may occur in one partner of a long and strongly bound marriage or in a union that is falling apart. Suffering from the loss of sexual function associated with some diseases will depend not only on the importance of sexual performance itself but also on its importance in the sick person's relationships.

A person is a political being. A person is in this sense equal to other persons, with rights and obligations and the ability to redress injury by others and the state. Sickness can interfere, producing the feeling of political powerlessness and lack of representation. Persons who are permanently handicapped may suffer from a feeling of exclusion from participation in the political realm.

Persons do things. They act, create, make, take apart, put together, wind, unwind, cause to be, and cause to vanish. They know themselves, and are known, by these acts. When illness restricts the range of activity of persons, they are not themselves.

Persons are often unaware of much that happens within them and why. Thus, there are things in the mind that cannot be brought to awareness by ordinary reflection. The structure of the unconscious is pictured quite differently by different scholars, but most students of human behavior accept the assertion that such an interior world exists. People can behave in ways that seem inexplicable and strange even to themselves, and the sense of powerlessness that the person may feel in the presence of such behavior can be a source of great distress.

Persons have regular behaviors. In health, we take for granted the details of our day-to-day behavior. Persons know themselves to be well as much by whether they behave as usual as by any other set of facts. Patients decide that they are ill because they cannot perform as usual, and they may suffer the loss of their routine. If they cannot do the things that they identify with the fact of their being, they are not whole.

Every person has a body. The relation with one's body may vary from identification with it to admiration, loathing, or constant fear. The body may even be perceived as a representation of a parent, so that when something happens to the person's body it is as though a parent were injured. Disease can so alter the relation that the body is no longer seen as a friend but, rather, as an untrustworthy enemy. This is intensified if the illness comes on without warning, and as illness persists, the person may feel increasingly vulnerable. Just as many people have an expanded sense of self as a result of changes in their bodies from exercise, the potential exists for a contraction of this sense through injury to the body.

Everyone has a secret life. Sometimes it takes the form of fantasies and dreams of glory; sometimes it has a real existence known to only a few. Within the secret life are fears, desires, love affairs of the past and present, hopes, and fantasies. Disease may destroy not only the public or the private person but the secret person, as well. A secret beloved friend may be lost to a sick person because he or she has no legitimate place by the sickbed. When that happens, the patient may have lost the part of life that made tolerable an otherwise embittered existence. Or the loss may be only of a dream, but one that might have come true. Such loss can be a source of great distress and intensely private pain.

Everyone has a perceived future. Events that one expects to come to pass vary from expectations for one's children to a belief in one's creative ability. Intense unhappiness results from a loss of the future—the future of the individual person, of children, and of other loved ones. Hope dwells in this dimension of existence, and great suffering attends the loss of hope.

Everyone has a transcendent dimension, a life of the spirit. This is most directly expressed in religion and the mystic traditions, but the frequency with which people have intense feelings of bonding with groups, ideals, or anything larger and more enduring than the person is evidence of the universality of the transcendent dimension. The quality of being greater and more lasting than an individual life gives this aspect of the person its timeless dimension. The profession of medicine appears to ignore the human spirit. When I see patients in nursing homes who have become only bodies, I wonder whether it is not their transcendent dimension that they have lost.

THE NATURE OF SUFFERING

For purposes of explanation, I have outlined various parts that make up a person. However, persons cannot be reduced to their parts in order to be better understood. Reductionist scientific methods, so successful in human biology, do not help us to comprehend whole persons. My intent was rather to suggest the complexity of the person and the potential for injury and suffering that exists in everyone. With this in mind, any suggestion of mechanical simplicity should disappear from my definition of suffering. All the aspects of personhood—the lived past, the family's lived past, culture and society, roles, the instrumental dimension, associations and relationships, the body, the unconscious mind, the political being, the secret life, the perceived future, and the transcendent dimension—are susceptible to damage and loss.

Injuries to the integrity of the person may be expressed by sadness, anger, loneliness, depression, grief, unhappiness, melancholy, rage, withdrawal, or yearning. We acknowledge the person's right to have and express such feelings. But we often forget that the affect is merely the outward expression of the injury, not the injury itself. We know little about the nature of the injuries themselves, and what we know has been learned largely from literature, not medicine.

If the injury is sufficient, the person suffers. The only way to learn what damage is sufficient to cause suffering, or whether suffering is present, is to ask the sufferer. We all recognize certain injuries that almost invariably cause suffering: the death or distress of loved ones, powerlessness, helplessness, hopelessness, torture, the loss of a life's work, betrayal, physical agony, isolation, homelessness, memory failure, and fear. Each is both universal and individual. Each touches features common to all of us, yet each contains features that must be defined in terms of a specific person at a specific time. With the relief of suffering in mind, however, we should reflect on how remarkably little is known of these injuries.

THE AMELIORATION OF SUFFERING

One might inquire why everyone is not suffering all the time. In a busy life, almost no day passes in which one's intactness goes unchallenged. Obviously, not every challenge is a threat. Yet I suspect that there is more suffering than is known. Just as people with chronic pain learn to keep it to themselves because others lose interest, so may those with chronic suffering.

There is another reason why every injury may not cause suffering. Persons are able to enlarge themselves in response to damage, so that instead of being reduced, they may indeed grow. This response to suffering has encouraged the belief that suffering is good for people. To some degree, and in some persons, this may be so. If a leg is injured so that an athlete cannot run again, the athlete may compensate for the loss by learning another sport or mode of expression. So it is with the loss of relationships, loves, roles, physical strength, dreams, and power. The human body may lack the capacity to gain a new part when one is lost, but the person has it.

The ability to recover from loss without succumbing to suffering is sometimes called resilience, as though nothing but elastic rebound were involved, but it is more as though an inner force were withdrawn from one manifestation of a person and redirected to another. If a child dies and the parent makes a successful recovery, the person is said to have "rebuilt" his or her life. The term suggests that the parts of the person are structured in a new manner, allowing expression in different dimensions. If a previously active person is confined to a wheelchair, intellectual pursuits may occupy more time.

Recovery from suffering often involves help, as though people who have lost parts of themselves can be sustained by the personhood of others until their own recovers. This is one of the latent functions of physicians: to lend strength. A group, too, may lend strength: Consider the success of groups of the similarly afflicted in easing the burden of illness (e.g., women with mastectomies, people with ostomies, and even the parents or family members of the afflicted).

Meaning and transcendence offer two additional ways by which the suffering associated with destruction of a part of personhood is ameliorated. Assigning a meaning to the injurious condition often reduces or even resolves the suffering associated with it. Most often, a cause for the condition is sought within past behaviors or beliefs. Thus, the pain or threat that causes suffering is seen as not destroying a part of the person, because it is part of the person by virtue of its origin within the self. In our culture, taking the blame for harm that comes to oneself because of the unconscious mind, serves the same purpose as the concept of karma in Eastern theologies; suffering is reduced when it can be located within a coherent set of meanings. Physicians are familiar with the question from the sick, "Did I do something that made this happen?" It is more tolerable for a terrible thing to happen because of something that one has done than it is to be at the mercy of chance.

Transcendence is probably the most powerful way in which one is restored to wholeness after an injury to personhood. When experienced, transcendence locates the person in a far larger landscape. The sufferer is not isolated by pain but is brought closer to a transpersonal source of meaning and to the human community that shares those meanings. Such an experience need not involve religion in any formal sense; however, in its transpersonal dimension, it is deeply spiritual. For example, patriotism can be a secular expression of transcendence.

WHEN SUFFERING CONTINUES

But what happens when suffering is not relieved? If suffering occurs when there is a threat to one's integrity or a loss of a part of a person, then suffering will continue if the person cannot be made whole again. Little is known about this aspect of suffering. Is much of what we call depression merely unrelieved suffering? Considering that depression commonly follows the loss of loved ones, business reversals, prolonged illness, profound injuries to self-esteem, and other damages to personhood, the possibility is real. In many chronic or serious diseases, persons who "recover" or who seem to be successfully treated do not return to normal function. They may never again be employed, recover sexual function, pursue career goals, reestablish family relationships, or reenter the social world, despite a physical cure. Such patients may not have recovered from the nonphysical changes occurring with serious illness. Consider the dimensions of personhood described above, and note that each is threatened or damaged in profound illness. It should come as no surprise, then, that chronic suffering frequently follows in the wake of disease.

The paradox with which this paper began—that suffering is often caused by the treatment of the sick—no longer seems so puzzling. How could it be otherwise, when medicine has concerned itself so little with the nature and causes of suffering? This lack is not a failure of good intentions. None are more concerned about pain or loss of function than physicians. Instead, it is a failure of knowledge and understanding. We lack knowledge, because in working from a dichotomy contrived within a historical context far from our own, we have artificially circumscribed our task in caring for the sick.

Attempts to understand all the known dimensions of personhood and their relations to illness and suffering present problems of staggering complexity. The problems are no greater, however, than those initially posed by the question of how the body works—a question that we have managed to answer in extraordinary detail. If the ends of medicine are to be directed toward the relief of human suffering, the need is clear.

AUTHOR NOTE

The author is indebted to Rabbi Jack Bemporad, Drs. Joan Cassell, Peter Dineen, Nancy McKenzie, Richard Zaner, Ms. Dawn McGuire, the members of the Research Group on Death, Suffering, and Well-Being of The Hastings Center for their advice and assistance, and to the Arthur Vining Davis Foundations for support of the research group.

REFERENCES

1. Cassell, E. "Being and Becoming Dead." *Soc Res.* 1972; 39: 528-42.

2. Bakan, D. *Disease, Pain and Sacrifice: Toward a Psychology of Suffering.* Chicago: Beacon Press, 1971.

3. Marks, R. M., Sachar, E.J. "Undertreatment of Medical Inpatients with Narcotic Analgesics." *Ann Intern Med.* 1973; 78: 173-81.

4. Kanner, R.M., Foley, K.M. "Patterns of Narcotic Drug Use in a Cancer Pain Clinic." *Ann NY Acad Sci.* 1981; 362: 161-72.

5. Goodwin, J.S., Goodwin, J.M., Vogel, A.V. "Knowledge and Use of Placebos by House Officers and Nurses." *Ann Intern Med.* 1979; 91: 106-10.

6. Zaner, R. *The Context Of Self: A Phenomenological Inquiry Using Medicine as a Clue.* Athens, Ohio: Ohio University Press, 1981.

The Role of the Social Worker on a Stroke Rehabilitation Unit

Judith M. Heller

I am a social worker on the Stroke Unit at Burke Rehabilitation Hospital. It is a 30 bed unit. Patients are mostly older adults with a variety of socioeconomic backgrounds, family situations and psychosocial needs. I work directly with the patients and their families in short-term counseling, helping them to adjust to the hospitalization, their disability, and to execute appropriate discharge plans.

THE INITIAL INTERVIEW

There are two social workers on our unit, and we meet with every patient and family or significant other. We first see them on the day they are admitted, to provide education and apply the "social" in social work. Historically, social workers were called "friendly visitors." Many times patients who are admitted are unsure of what a rehabilitation hospital is. They are frightened, and may think they are in a nursing home and will never be able to return to their own homes. My colleague and I explain the program to them, describe briefly what occupational therapy, physical therapy and speech therapy involve, and inform them of their approximate length of stay.

Judith M. Heller, MSW, CSW, is currently specializing in the Stroke Unit at the Burke Rehabilitation Hospital. Prior to this she was a supervisor of clinical social work, at Columbia and Fordham Universities, in New York City.

[Haworth co-indexing entry note]: "The Role of the Social Worker on a Stroke Rehabilitation Unit." Heller, Judith M. Co-published simultaneously in *Loss, Grief & Care* (The Haworth Press, Inc.) Vol. 8, No. 1/2, 1998, pp. 143-147; and: *After Stroke: Enhancing Quality of Life* (ed: Wallace Sife) The Haworth Press, Inc., 1998, pp. 143-147. Single or multiple copies of this article are available for a fee from The Haworth Document Delivery Service [1-800-342-9678, 9:00 a.m. - 5:00 p.m. (EST). E-mail address: getinfo@haworth.com].

Gathering a social history is also a part of this initial interview. Knowing a patient's background will help, not only in our planning for the patient's future, but will also help other members of the team to work more effectively. The information gathered covers, among other things, languages spoken, birth place, names of family members as well as employment history, hobbies, and general life style. We try to draw as complete a picture as we can of the patient, prior to the event, and use that information in our work. As an example, Mr. X, a 53 year old, born in Haiti, came to New York when he was three years old. His wife knows him as only English speaking; yet the speech therapist reports he is speaking gibberish. But the gibberish sounds a little like French. Given he was born in Haiti, a French speaking island, we enlisted an interpreter who told us the patient was, indeed, speaking French. Another example: Mr. A. was not motivated to attend physical therapy but was known to be an avid golfer. Physical therapy sessions were moved out onto the grass, a golf club was incorporated into his treatment and, the patient then faithfully attended all his program sessions.

The family dynamics, the interaction between the patient and family, and the family with each other is also valuable information. We make note of the emotional and physical condition of the spouse and of his or her ability to understand the patient's deficits. Does the family make excuses for the patient's inability to respond (i.e., He is tired now. He doesn't like to speak with strangers. He moved his arm for me, yesterday.)? Are they in denial?

At some point in this interview we address those people who will be involved in the patient's long range discharge plans. They are told about our policy to observe a therapeutic program, and of our interest in training the caregiver.

COUNSELING

Providing supportive counseling to the patients and their families is one of the primary roles of the social worker on the unit. We meet with each patient at least one time per week, and their families or significant others as needed.

Patients and their families experience much of the same stages of mourning, described by Elizabeth Kubler-Ross in her book *On Death and Dying*: denial, anger, bargaining, depression and acceptance. The angry patient may lack motivation and refuse to co-operate with the therapists, or attend the program. The depressed patient may be labile much of the time, and express fear about the future. He will have fears about being able to resume his former lifestyle and return to work, travel, sports, etc. He may also be preoccupied with the fear that he will have another stroke and be a burden to his family. It is important for the patient to work through, understand and ventilate his feelings.

For some couples, marital counseling is appropriate, before the patient and spouse go home. They need to be open with each other in discussing issues on sexuality and living with a disability. We counsel them in this, also.

The most frazzled group we deal with are those family members known as the "sandwich generation." They are adults who have children of their own and now find they must become decision-maker and caretaker to their parents. They feel caught in the middle. We have found that besides individual counseling, support groups are helpful to these families. We have an educational support group which is interdisciplinary, and facilitated by the social worker. Each week a different team member presents for one-half hour, and the social worker speaks the second half hour, dealing with the emotional issues and concerns of the group.

SOCIAL WORK AND THE TEAM APPROACH

On our Stroke Unit at Burke Rehabilitation Hospital we work closely as a team, to share information about each patient. It is my role, as social worker, to know how the patient is doing and be the liaison between him, his family, and the rest of our staff. I also want to know how a caregiver manages with the patient during training sessions, so a safe discharge plan can be formulated. In most of the cases the worker will organize a family-team conference involving the caregiver and family members. This is a forum in which we can discuss the patient's condition, needs and prognosis.

All of the patient's activities are based on the Stroke Unit. At any time during the day, we can watch the patient in his activities, and be an active part of the treatment. Being able to see the patient's actual status helps in counseling him, and enables us to be available to the therapists, in the event of a problem.

DISCHARGING THE PATIENT

Discharging a patient is an interdisciplinary decision. All team members have input and must answer the question "Has the patient reached a plateau, or achieved his/her goals?" If yes, then a discharge date is set, giving the patient and family a two-week notice. In some cases, the patient's insurance coverage or the insurance carrier's case manager will determine the date.

As we have previously noted, the family members are asked to attend training programs. Not only do we ask them to come to occupational, physical and speech therapies, but if the worker feels the caregiver needs to learn the patient's total care needs, we will arrange for that person to sleep over, in the patient's room. He/she is asked to follow the routine of early morning care, and respond to late night needs (in some cases, learning tube feeding, catheterization, and administering insulin). At this point in time, the worker can discuss the caregiver's feelings about doing these tasks, and whether or not he/she feels the patient can be managed at home. Many times this program will help convince caregivers that they need to get private help, or that the patient needs more care than they can provide, and nursing home placement may be a better plan for them.

Most patients are entitled to some type of home care or outpatient program after they leave the hospital setting. The social worker will discuss options with the team and patient and family, and make any referrals, accordingly. We will also direct them to resources available in the community, such as Meals-On-Wheels, Lifeline, and transportation and other support groups.

We have to keep in mind that being discharged from the hospital is stressful for the stroke patient, as well as for his family. This represents a termination of intense involvement with the people who were providing a strong measure of security and hope.

We sometimes find that families in denial, who have had the mistaken belief that the patient would regain total functioning by discharge, will resist leaving. They lose all hope, and are afraid the stroke survivor will not get any better. Some feel rejected by the team ("You're putting us out too soon" or "You've given up on me").

This makes discharge a stressful time for those of us providing the care, as well. We, as social workers, must lend support to the team and work together, in dealing with these frustrations. The patients and families are being confronted with the realities of the disabilities, the responsibilities involved, and uncertainties about their future. They may be having problems coping, so they tend to place the blame on us.

As a team we have to be in touch with our own feelings about the patient's discharge. We have to communicate openly, in order to assure a coordinated approach to each patient and family, in their adjustment to going home and on to the next step.

In conclusion, the role of the social worker on the Stroke Rehabilitation Unit is to handle the practical and educational discharge issues, as well as to provide social and emotional support for the patients and their families. We also offer insight and supportiveness to our team members, help to work out the best approach to patient relations, and provide them with a constructive outlet to vent their feelings.

PART III
PERSONAL REFLECTIONS

Stroke!
This Isn't the Script I Was Writing!

Barbara Vance

My favorite philosopher, Ziggy, says in one of his cartoons, "If all the world is a stage and we are merely players, how come I get only bit parts?" Bit parts or not, I'm glad to be playing on this giant stage called the world. For a while I didn't even know I was part of that giant stage. Lots of bit players in my own personal stroke drama left of center stage made it possible for me to play all those bit parts Ziggy is so concerned about.

My friend and favorite contemporary author, Madeleine L'Engle goes beyond Ziggy's idea in her poem, *Act III, Scene ii*:

Someone has altered the script
My lines have been changed.
The other actors are shifting roles.

Barbara Vance, PhD, is Professor of Family Sciences and Psychology at Brigham Young University.

[Haworth co-indexing entry note]: "Stroke! This Isn't the Script I Was Writing!." Vance, Barbara. Co-published simultaneously in *Loss, Grief & Care* (The Haworth Press, Inc.) Vol. 8, No. 1/2, 1998, pp. 149-160; and: *After Stroke: Enhancing Quality of Life* (ed: Wallace Sife) The Haworth Press, Inc., 1998, pp. 149-160. Single or multiple copies of this article are available for a fee from The Haworth Document Delivery Service [1-800-342-9678, 9:00 a.m. - 5:00 p.m. (EST). E-mail address: getinfo@haworth.com].

They don't come on when they're expected to,
and they don't say the lines I've written
and I'm being upstaged.
I thought I was writing this play
with a rather nice role for myself,
small, but juicy
and some excellent lines.
But nobody gives my cues
and the scenery has been replaced.
I don't recognize the new sets.
This isn't the script I was writing.
I don't understand this plot at all.

To grow up
is to find
the small part you are playing
in this extraordinary drama
written by
somebody else.

I guess I've grown up because I've discovered I'm playing a small part in an extraordinary drama written by somebody else. I've discovered this isn't the script I was writing, at all. And that's okay.

Playing a small part does not mean it is an unimportant one. However, we must admit that, though we are the main characters in our own life dramas, we also are playing very important bit parts in a larger drama. Some of us get stage fright and want out of this play we're in. Some of us play our parts well. Others don't play them well, at all.

Each day of my life I'm handed only the pages of the script for that day. Sometimes I can't read the script very well. Sometimes I don't want to play what is written in the script. But I have no idea how this drama I'm in will end. I'm in it up to my neck, now. I want to know how it will end. And I have a feeling if I don't play my part to the hilt, this drama won't end the way the writer expects it to.

MY STORY

I will describe to you a portion of a playlet that took place, perhaps left of center stage, in which I am the central character. The portion I will describe is more dramatic than most such playlets, but I didn't write the script. I'll just describe to you what happened as the script was written by somebody else. You might try to imagine yourself writing this. Could you ever in your wildest imagination come up with such a script? But remember, I'm not writing this script. I'm just describing.

I am a professor at Brigham Young University (BYU). I went to Israel in January 1986 on sabbatical leave, for a semester, to work as a visiting scholar at the University of Haifa. During my leave I lived at the home of Israeli friends, on Mt. Carmel, in Haifa.

End of semester final examinations at the University of Haifa started the week after I arrived. There was a three-week break between semesters, following final exams. Rather than accepting an invitation from Israeli colleagues to go with them to Kenya on a photographic safari, I decided to use the semester break to remain at the university and work on some research I had started with another colleague there.

Four days before the end of the semester break I took a bus from Haifa to Jerusalem, where I had made arrangements to stay at the guest house of Kibbutz Ramat Rachel, in south Jerusalem, where our BYU Study Abroad program was then located. Our new BYU Jerusalem Center for Near Eastern Studies was being constructed on Mt. Scopus, immediately south of Hebrew University. During those four days I visited the construction site of our new center, and arranged with the administrators for a world conference on the family to be conducted there, two years after construction was completed. I visited former students who were then in the Study-Abroad program, and walked all over the new and old cities of Jerusalem, the day before returning to the Haifa sites I had visited 10 years earlier, when I was a tourist in Israel.

It was Monday morning, February 10, 1986, the day I was to return to Haifa. Rain had fallen intermittently during my four-day sojourn in Jerusalem, but this particular morning dawned beautiful sunshine. For some reason, however, I had a very difficult time rising from my bed and getting myself ready for the two-and-a-half-hour bus trip to Haifa.

I couldn't find the central bus station, and I was becoming more and more tired and agitated. Fortunately, a bit player in my little drama, an Arab woman, stopped to give me assistance. She couldn't speak English and I couldn't speak Arabic. Eventually she grabbed my hand and literally led me to the bus station, which was just around the corner. I just had not gone far enough to see the back of the station. Lo and behold, there, in its stall was my bus to Haifa. I purchased my ticket and climbed aboard. The front seat was empty so I decided to sit there.

As I lifted my suitcase and my loaded bookpack onto the seat beside me, I felt a cracking sensation across the back of my neck. I thought I had pulled a muscle, while lifting the bags to the seat. I rubbed my neck and shoulder muscles, but that didn't seem to help. I also felt very ill. I couldn't figure out what was wrong with me. I remember thinking that I didn't have anything better to do, so I slumped down into my window seat and decided to relax on the bus for that long ride back to Haifa.

I didn't know it at the time, but a congenital aneurysm had burst in the base of my brain, when I thought I had pulled a muscle. My brain was being flooded with a massive hemorrhage. Blood, when it flows where it isn't supposed to, is very toxic to body tissue. That hemorrhage was what was making me feel so ill. My surgeons told me much later, when I left the hospital, that I should have been dead within seconds, if not minutes, after the bursting of the aneurysm. There is no medical explanation for my survival of that massive hemorrhage—the most lethal kind of stroke.

When the bus arrived in the Haifa central bus station, I had a world-class headache. I was still feeling awful, but the headache was so intense it almost made me forget how awful I felt. I decided I should get a cab instead of a city bus up to Mt. Carmel, where I was living with my Israeli family.

But when I got out to the curb at the bus station, there was my bus to Mt. Carmel. Like a fool, I climbed aboard and hobbled with my bags to the place in the back, where people can stand with their luggage. For the next half hour I managed to keep my bags in place while the bus climbed the switchback road maze up to Mt. Carmel. I rang the buzzer for my stop, but when the bus stopped I could not manage to get out of my seat and get my bags off the bus. The door closed and the bus lurched on to the next stop more than a half-mile away. I yelled, "Regal, Regal!" (Hebrew for "wait a minute") to the driver, but only a whisper came out. That was one sign of stroke, by the way.

At the next stop I was able to get my bags off the bus. I tied them to a luggage carrier I had with me and pulled them behind me three-quarters of a mile before I reached the end of a cul de sac, where 155 steps led down to just a block from home.

But I became so nauseated at the end of the cul de sac that I started to look around for a place to throw up. Leaving my bags at the top of the stairway, I found a stairwell leading down to an apartment building. When I reached the point of dry heaves, I took off my coat (it had been chilly in Jerusalem, but it was hot in Haifa), threw it over the stair wall and slumped down on a step, leaning against my coat.

I knew people were passing by on the stairway, and probably even staring at me, but I didn't care. It seemed too bright for me to open my eyes. So I closed them. I couldn't focus them anyway (another sign of stroke!). Suddenly I realized I was losing consciousness. Another bit player, who must have been a Jewish Israeli woman (remember I couldn't open my eyes and focus them), who could speak flawless English, sat down next to me, and asked how she could help. I told her my name and the telephone number of the apartment. I told her to go immediately and call because I was losing consciousness. I never saw that woman again. She was only a bit player in my little drama, but she saved my life.

A few minutes later I heard the screech of car brakes and then footsteps coming in my direction. Hedy, the mother in the family I was living with, rushed to my side. She put her arms around me and told me that an ambulance was on its way and that her daughter, who was then a student in the high school, was on her way over by foot. They wanted to make sure they wouldn't miss me.

When the girl got to us and caught her breath, she and her mother helped me to the car. I guess I looked more ill than they originally thought, and they decided not to wait for the ambulance. I slumped into the back seat of the car. Carmel Hospital was less than a mile away.

When the car arrived at the emergency entrance to the hospital, the ER personnel knew immediately that I had suffered a stroke, but they didn't know what kind. I remember the doors on either side of the car opening, hands reaching for me, voices speaking in agitated Hebrew. But most of all, I remember being more fatigued than I had ever felt in my life. I wanted to sleep.

I felt everything would be okay, now, so I went to sleep. Actually, I had lost consciousness. What I know about the next three weeks in my life was described to me after I was released from the hospital. I have only a few disconnected memories of that three-week period in the hospital. My Israeli family took charge of everything, from then on. More bit players–but so very important in my little drama.

Carmel Hospital does not have a neurological service. But Rambam Hospital, just a 20-minute ride away, on the shore of the Mediterranean Sea, does. So emergency preparations were arranged for me to be taken there by ambulance. But on the way, in that ambulance, I died. My vital signs stopped. My brain had imploded on my brain stem, stopping my breathing and heartbeat. The medical technicians in the ambulance could not revive me.

When I arrived at Rambam Hospital, three neurosurgeons, who also are professors in the medical school at the Technion in Haifa, were waiting for me. Dr. Levy quickly drilled into my skull to release the pressure of the hemorrhage on my brain. That was the first surgery. It brought back my vital signs.

Thirty hours later, following a whole series of tests, I was wheeled into surgery for a 10-hour marathon by Drs. Feinsod, Levy, and Berkowitz, to snip out nine aneurysms ready to blow, and resect the blood vessels in the base of my brain near the cerebellum. All my hair had been shaved off for that second surgery. When I left, my head was shrouded in bandages. My Israeli family and friends from Jerusalem, waiting for me to come out of the recovery room, said that when I appeared, I was "unrecognizable." I had survived the long surgery, but would I survive the next few critical days? A patient after such a procedure can survive the surgery but die because of subsequent swelling of the brain, because of the skull confinement.

I was lucky. I survived those 10 days in ICU, as well as another 11 days in the neurosurgical ward, which I shared mostly with Arab, and a few Jewish, survivors of neurosurgery.

I don't remember bandages on my head at all. As a matter of fact, I had a terrible time comprehending that I had had brain surgery. Because no member of my family from the States could get to Israel right away, my many colleagues and friends in Israel, including some I had never met before my stroke, and the members of our little congregation in Jerusalem, visited me daily to keep me awake and alert. When my brain had imploded on my brain stem, that part of the brain stem that controls the ability to go to sleep and wake up and remain attentive was severely damaged. That meant I had to have visitors to keep me awake. I was told there were over 100 such bit players, while I lay for three weeks in my bed at Rambam Hospital. I don't remember most of them, but they literally saved my life.

Following stabilization of vital signs, rehabilitation usually begins after a stroke. Rambam did not have a rehabilitation unit, but Hadassa Hospital in Jerusalem did. However, there were no beds available. So I remained at Rambam until other arrangements could be made for my care when I left the hospital. I went to Jerusalem to the apartment of a family in our congregation. The mother is a registered nurse. At the time, I needed round-the-clock nursing.

Ten days after I left Rambam Hospital, my sister from Idaho and her husband arrived to accompany me back home. My health was good enough at the time, so they were able to spend a few extra days, touring the country with the father of the family I was staying with. He was a travel guide.

Now, I have celebrated eight years since my stroke. I returned to work at BYU, four months after that episode! That probably wasn't a very wise thing to do. I didn't realize at the time how much I still had to do, to recover. I felt I had been hit by a Mack truck and couldn't figure out why I couldn't get my strength and stamina back. The stroke completely destroyed my center of balance, so I walked with help and a definite tilt to the right, undoubtedly looking most of the time like a drunken sailor. I accomplished in five weeks of physical therapy what normally would have taken at least five months, and more likely much longer. I was determined to get back to normal, whatever that was. I had to wait an awfully long time for my brain to heal, and new nerve connections to be established. But there could be no new nerve cells, because I had all I was ever going to get, at birth.

As a result of the stroke, I lost 30 pounds, which I couldn't afford to lose at the time. I would tell people I had morning sickness without the reward at the end of nine months! All my nausea cells in the base of my brain had been damaged by the stroke. Strangely enough, that nausea lasted exactly nine months. In the meantime, I had a terrible time eating anything. But I slowly gained back the weight I had lost.

Today I'm about 90 percent back to normal, with my balance and appetite back in fine form. It took many, many months of determination and sheer guts, lots of prayer and a miracle to get where I am today. But I wouldn't be alive now, or as well as I am, without hundreds of bit players in my little drama, left of center stage. Not one of these bit players upstaged anyone else. Otherwise, it wouldn't have worked.

WHAT I HAVE LEARNED ABOUT RECOVERY

To see me now, you would never guess that I had experienced anything so physically traumatic. Before that, had I been writing the script of my life, I would have left out the stroke. But not now. My experience in recovery has taught me some very important lessons about this "drama being written by somebody else." I learned several invaluable lessons about recovery and about thriving, not just surviving.

1. I learned that once in recovery, always in recovery. My disabilities are silent, invisible ones, but I know they are there. Though I no longer walk with canes, when the moon is full I struggle with my balance. (I think it's a gravity kind of thing.) When there is an eclipse of the sun or the moon I almost go crazy. The balance thing again. Little things still irritate me. I've learned that these little inconveniences are part of my recovery and that I'll probably always struggle with them, now and then.

I live with recurring post-traumatic stress disorder or PTSD, commonly known as shell shock. I've never been in combat. However, I have flashbacks and fears undoubtedly related to my stroke. At times they are gut-wrenching and so frightening as almost to paralyze me, just as during the weeks immediately following my stroke. My PTSD isn't nearly as frequent now, or as extreme. But it comes and goes. I've learned to recognize it and accept it as a part of me, as something that happens less and less often now. I can't change it. No amount of therapy can help it go away. Somehow, it is easier when I accept it and recognize that it will be back, again. I'll not fight it the way I once did. It is a part of my life I can't change.

2. I've learned to live with little irritations that sometimes can become "tremendous trifles." It was terribly difficult for me to recognize that part of recovery from stroke is learning to live with unusual sensitivity and irritation with little things, such as some noises and sights and even feelings. I've learned, as with PTSD, to simply accept these little irritations as part of me. I can't change them, although things that would have irritated me so keenly in the months following my stroke no longer have the same intense effect.

3. I have learned how much I need other people. After my stroke I lost some friends, but they usually turned out to be the "do things with" kind of friends. I can't run anymore, and am unable to play tennis, so there go my tennis friends. I love to sing, but I can't sing in trios or quartets, or even solo as I once did, because of the tracheotomy tube down my throat during that long surgery. My singing voice is gone, but I still use it. There is an old saw, "Use it or lose it." I sang with others, and it was a wonderful social outlet. And it still is, in spite of the fact I can't do what I once did. My real singing friends understand what I now can and can't do, and that I still appreciate harmony. I still give it a good try, though, even if I'm not as successful as I once was.

Yes, I need other people. Though I can't do some things I once did, that doesn't mean I can get through life alone. I need others—my family, my friends. I need them and they need me. The nature of relationships changes through the years, as it should. I am dynamic, and so are the people in my life. This unpredictable diversity in relationships is challenging and necessary.

4. I've learned to stop and smell the roses along the way. My stroke was caused by the bursting of a congenital aneurysm. There really isn't anything I could have done about it. I didn't display any of the symptoms that would have predicted a stroke. It was unavoidable. When the blood vessels in my brain were old enough, and thus thin enough, one of the 10 aneurysms in my brain burst, causing the hemorrhage, and the stroke.

I was very fortunate. In order to recover I simply had to slow down. I had been accustomed to doing everything quickly—yesterday, if possible! But in this process of recovery, I discovered I had been passing up much of the best of life. I was allowing things that matter the least to seem to matter most. I've learned to allow myself to take a day off, now and then. I've learned to pay more attention to the people around me, and to enjoy conversations with them, even lingering ones that I didn't allow myself before my stroke. I'm paying more attention to the changing seasons around me.

I live in a desert valley, surrounded by beautiful mountains. Now I am appreciating the beauty here, as never before. I don't take work home with me in my briefcase. I do what I can do at the office in a day. Then when I leave work, I take my head home with me, as well as my heart. I leave my work back at the office. I enjoy to the hilt my evening hours, and weekends.

At one time I used to work through my vacation periods every year, because I had so much to do—books to write, articles to write, class preparations to make. But no more! When it is vacation time, I take a real vacation. I clear the inevitable cobwebs out of my head, so when I return to work I'm refreshed and renewed.

I've also learned to be a kid, again. Children are naturally good at living in the moment and having fun. I always thought I had fun before. But now that I've learned to be a kid again, having fun now is a whole new ball game.

But to be quite frank, I keep tending to return to the fast lane again. Every once in a while I have to remind myself to slow down and smell the roses. I've learned that taking time to slow down, to appreciate all the beauty around me, is worth it.

5. I've learned to accept what I can't change. I think perhaps I've spent too much of my life attempting to break down walls that were too thick to penetrate. No more. I'm much better at recognizing and accepting what I can't change, and I don't waste my time anymore complaining about them. I just go on with something I can change. I've learned to let things go. Life is too short.

6. I've learned to play the cards I'm dealt. Sometimes I get the feeling that the world I'm living in is going to Hades in a handbasket—fast. However, I live in this world. It's the only one I know. I'll do what I can to create a good one, right here, where I live.

Lots of things I can't control occur in my life—such as my stroke. But those are the cards I was dealt at the time. Instead of berating what happened to me, I figured out how to get better and better, all the time. Now, I do that with any challenge in life. I decide how to cope with it. Sometimes

I do a terrific job with stroke recovery, and sometimes I do a terrible job. But each day I do what I can, and do that as best as I know how. And that's all that's necessary. I take what comes, change what I can–the best I can. And I let the rest go.

7. I've learned to be more patient, which has never been one of my virtues. I've learned this primarily in my work with children (I'm a child psychologist and therapist), and in playing the violin. Children do not do things according to my time scale. But I've discovered a whole new world by patiently looking at the world through the eyes of a child. It's a fascinating world full of wonder. Playing the violin, which is not by any means easy, has also taught me to be patient with the slow progress of skill development and the creation of beautiful music.

Recovery from a stroke has reinforced the patience I've learned from working with children and playing the violin. I discovered that the human body is a magnificent thing. But that splendid organism must have the time it needs to recover. I thought my stroke recovery would take just a few months. No way. It has taken much longer, and I'm still in recovery. I'm not where I was in the beginning, and I'm not where I will be years down the road. I am lucky, and most of my former skills have returned. But now I have lots of fine-tuning to do.

8. I've learned to let go and get on with my life. During the first year, following my stroke, I probably drove people crazy, talking about my stroke. One day about 10 months into recovery, one of my dear friends said to me, "You're not your stroke, you know!" That brought me up short. And I did a lot of thinking about what she meant. She was tired of hearing me talk about my stroke. She missed the conversations we once enjoyed that were not about my stroke. I think such constant talking about that subject was my way of coming to terms with what had happened to me. It was a stage I had to go through.

But I'm not my stroke. I'm Barbara. Although there are a few people in my life who still define me by my stroke, I'll just have to let that be their problem. In the meantime, I've let my stroke go. Now I'm into another stage of my life.

I've discovered that life is really a long series of letting-go experiences. I let go of my parental family when I left to live on my own. I let go of my graduate studies at Stanford (which were beautiful, but very tough years in my life). I let go of living in another part of the country, in order to reside where I am now–and on and on. This doesn't mean I've let go of beautiful memories. I hang on to wonderful memories, let bad memories go, and get on with my life. Every once in a while I have to remind myself to let something go, and get on with my life. I'm getting better and better by the day, at letting go. I don't need excess baggage from the past, controlling my present.

9. I've learned to live in the moment. As a child psychologist, I've learned from children that every moment counts. I would tell myself in graduate school that someday I'll do such-and-such. But Ph.D. sometimes means "piled higher and deeper." It took my stroke to force me to recognize that now is the only time there is. There is the past; and it is gone, so I can't do anything about it. There is the future, but it isn't here yet. Living in the moment like a child, and enjoying it, is something I've learned as a result of my recovery from stroke. And I've learned to laugh while I am enjoying the moment. There is the child in me that wants to get out, all the time. And I let that child out a lot, these days.

10. I've learned to do what I'm really interested in, and gifted at. It has taken me many years to learn that I can't do everything as well as I would like. I've never been satisfied with anything but perfection. But I've never achieved perfection in anything, mainly because my criteria for this keep getting more numerous as I go along.

My stroke forced me to take a long, cold look at what I'm doing in this world. I've had my share of successes, and also my share of failures. But I've decided to take control of my own life, thanks to my stroke. I say no to lots of things I could do, mainly because I'm not *really* interested in whatever it is and, I don't feel any particular gift in that area. I don't want to spend the rest of my life in the thick of thin things. I want to focus my limited energies and time on those things I have some gifts for doing, and am really interested in. If what I do doesn't please others, at least it will please me. But I think, given my past experience with this one, that what I do accomplish, enriches not only my life, but the lives of others.

Now, consider all the bit players (real important) in this little playlet I've just described, left of center stage, where I am the central character. What would have happened if the Arab woman in Jerusalem hadn't come along to help me find the bus to Haifa? What would have happened if the Jewish woman had not recognized my desperate need for help on Mt. Carmel, in Haifa? What would have happened if my Israeli family had not been home when the call for help came? What would have happened if my neurosurgeons had not been available at Rambam Medical Center? What would have happened if my Israeli friends and the students in our Study-Abroad program hadn't visited me in the hospital? And I haven't even mentioned the many here in the States, especially the members of my family. I am not aware of any bit player who opted out of his or her role in my little playlet.

But most important of all, I've learned how connected we all are to each other. I work in a "publish-or-perish" profession. However, I've learned that my most important work is not what I write about, or what I research, but how I relate to others. I am connected to each person on this planet. Some cross my path not at all. Some for a moment only. Some lots of times. But whatever the case, we all are irrevocably connected. My greatest work is to serve and to love. I deeply believe we are all on a common journey. My work is to support each person I meet on that journey. My work is to love unconditionally. Shakespeare said each of us plays many roles in our lifetime. Some of those roles have many lines. Some only a few. Some are only walk-on roles.

We are not always patted on the back for the roles we play. Those often involve service to others–lots of it. We serve because something inside us impels us in a unique way toward our fellow human beings–our fellow travelers in this journey of life. Most deserve our service. Some do not. But we are not scorekeepers. We are servants. We are playing important roles in the larger drama of life–that extraordinary central drama, the script for which is being written by someone else. That drama is full of people we know and people we don't know. But we are all brothers and sisters and, therefore, inextricably connected to one another.

REFERENCE

L'Engle, M. (1978). Act III, Scene ii. In *The Weather of the Heart*. Wheaton, IL: Harold Shaw, Publishers.

AHA!
There Is a Reason

Casey Shannon

As we begin the long and difficult journey of recovery from a life-threatening illness or loss, one of our first thoughts is, "Why me?" Can there possibly be some reason? I am reminded of the wise and mysterious words spoken by my grandmother, when I was a young child. I can still hear her say, "Casey, for every event that takes place in our lives, there is a reason. There is a reason, even if we can't see clearly, and are unable to lift the dark veil of confusion that sometimes covers our eyes." I remember hearing her poignant words, and then conveniently forgetting them–until an event occurred in my life which completely changed my world.

At the productive and exciting age of 36, I experienced a massive brain-stem stroke. At that time I was happily married with a beautiful 13 year old daughter just starting high school. I was engaged in a thriving career as a high school art teacher, and also as a freelance artist. In addition, I was an avid skier, and felt as if I was flying high on top of the world. Who could ask for more?

The prognosis for my stroke recovery was not good, at that time. I was unable to breathe, swallow, or speak. In addition, the right side of my body was completely paralyzed. To make matters even worse, I was right-handed and needed that hand to draw. However, I worked very hard in my rehabilitation, even adding programs and drawing on personal resources that I intuitively knew would assist me in my recovery. I am delighted to report that I have experienced a wonderful recovery, even though I have

Casey Shannon, BFA, MS, is an academic and career Counselor at Cabrillo College Disabled Student Services, Stroke Center, and Women's Center.

[Haworth co-indexing entry note]: "AHA! There Is a Reason." Shannon, Casey. Co-published simultaneously in *Loss, Grief & Care* (The Haworth Press, Inc.) Vol. 8, No. 1/2, 1998, pp. 161-164; and: *After Stroke: Enhancing Quality of Life* (ed: Wallace Sife) The Haworth Press, Inc., 1998, pp. 161-164. Single or multiple copies of this article are available for a fee from The Haworth Document Delivery Service [1-800-342-9678, 9:00 a.m. - 5:00 p.m. (EST). E-mail address: getinfo@haworth.com].

not regained total control of my body. But I have since learned that regaining control is not what recovery is all about.

It was not until I reached a certain delicate balance between physical control and mental awareness that I began to genuinely appreciate my grandmother's loving words. Time went on, and as I lived my new life, a new wisdom grew with me. I now know that in addition to trying to understand the underlying reasons for the events in our lives, ultimately, each of us must learn them for ourselves. Hopefully, we will be able to derive some meaning from our searching.

After living with and adapting to the effects of my stroke for the past eleven years, I have finally come to realize the profound purpose of it all. The universe has placed me where I am today, to continue as an educator–a very special kind of educator. That is not a person who has a classroom with four walls, textbooks, seats, lesson plans and students. I mean an educator who educates the world–every person he/she comes in contact with, each day. And this responsibility falls especially on those of us who have experienced major disability and hardship.

Over the past eleven years, I have been confronted, time and time again, by people who "haven't got a clue" about the real lives and feelings of others. This situation even extends to those individuals who claim to be sensitive and compassionate. But, try as they may, these people can't really understand. The bottom line here is, if you don't have a disability, you can't really know what it is like. You may gain some knowledge, awareness or even a tolerance for this, but you can never truly understand it. There is an old saying that captures the essence of this, "There is no way of knowing without experiencing."

After re-entering college for graduate school, and later earning a master's degree, I am currently considered to be a professional woman, again. Now I am a counselor and the co-director of a women's center at a California community college. In my profession and daily routines I encounter many different kinds of people who are dealing with their own agendas–to the point of being submerged in them. When people are so preoccupied with their own issues, they are likely to be insensitive or even oblivious to that which does not directly concern them. Typically, many people go through their days with this perpetual lack of perspective–or even some state of denial or wishful thinking. I will not deny that, at times, I also have fallen victim, under this dark veil of confusion.

There was a time when encounters with "clueless" people really bothered me. Occasionally, these confrontations would corrode my sense of self-esteem, which I had worked so hard to recapture after my stroke. I am sure that those "clueless" encounters with other people were not intended to hurt me. They just happened and I reacted. Here are a few examples of some typical encounters I have experienced.

1. People walking or bumping into me and knocking me over.
2. People shouting during ordinary conversation, because they think I am blind, I can't hear, or I don't understand.
3. When entering a busy building, people slamming doors in my face.
4. People pushing, in their haste to get to their destinations.
5. Attending my 30th high school reunion, but now being ignored by many of my former classmates.
6. When I am out to dinner, the waiter or waitress asks others in my party what she (meaning me) would like to order.

At work, the encounters continue, under the guise of professionalism or constructive criticism:

7. Co-workers questioning me why I have to be so formal and type everything on a computer (even quick little notes) and accusing me of wasting time. (Using a Computer is much easier for me than writing with my non-dominant hand.)
8. There was an E-mail message for me from an English teacher, criticizing my use of all CAPS, when sending a campus communication. (That is quicker and easier for me, when typing with one hand).
9. After meetings, most fellow faculty members will gather up their things and rush out the door. While talking in groups they ignore and leave me behind.

In instances like these, I used to allow myself to be hurt, frustrated, and feel less than whole. I was left with my insecurities, wondering about my worth as a person. And I would doubt my personal value, and question my place in the world. It took many painful encounters with others for me to eventually realize that this was not my problem. It was *their* problem, caused by lack of knowledge or understanding of disabilities. But whatever the cause, I should not make it my trouble.

I slowly began to realize it was my responsibility to firmly and politely confront people in these situations. Instead of reacting negatively or being defensively silent, what was needed was for me to speak up. At first, I timidly put this idea into action. To my surprise I was rewarded, as many actually showed a willingness to acquire an awareness about my position, as I explained my needs to them. When I realized what was happening, the "world educator" concept shot into my mind. It ripped the dark veil of confusion from my eyes and offered me the answer. My buried thoughts shouted to me, "Of course, that's it!" I realized that if I don't stop and take the time to educate others about people with disabilities, and teach them about understanding, tolerance, and compassion, who will? My entire being exploded with a joyous realization. So, this was what my wise grandmother had been talking about! This was what I had been searching for and struggling to understand.

Actually, if you stop and think about it, everybody has some degree of "cluelessness" concerning the lives of others. This might be about disability, disease and illness, racial diversity, cultural tradition, substance abuse, addiction, or religious beliefs to name only a few. As my grandmother used to say, "We can't walk in another person's shoes." It makes sense to accept that everyone on this earth could benefit from a little understanding, tolerance and compassion. Each of us can make some difference in helping improve someone else's life.

In our sometimes threatening and difficult life situations, there is a tiny thread of commonalty that weaves our experiences together. This thread is made up of our human feelings of despair, loss, survival and hope–to name a few. These shared emotions are the foundation for our having empathy for each other. But we first have to choose to take responsibility for our newly discovered awareness. Only then can we really begin to do something about it.

I like to think of this as an extended metaphor. If, indeed, we have chosen wisely, two strong and bright threads appear in our consciousness, ready for our careful weaving. One brilliant thread of commonalty and one luminous thread of awareness can be woven together to create the fabric of a marvelous cape, which can shelter us and enrich all of our lives. Embraced in the warm folds of this wrap, we can open the sometimes smudged window of tolerance and allow a soothing breeze of understanding to gently caress our spirit.

Isn't life wonderful and amazing? But sometimes even the simplest of concepts elude us. Thank goodness we never stop searching and learning! If we work hard at it, and make it so, the stroke experience can be just the beginning of a new and marvelous life.

The Words I Lost

Abraham H. Raskin

As the national labor correspondent of *The New York Times* for over 40 years, and frequent contributor to the *New Yorker, Fortune, Forbes* and other leading publications, I have always considered a vibrant, principled and purposeful union movement a hallmark of American democracy. My mission, I felt, was to bridge together organized labor, the employers, the workers and the government.

My most valuable tool, I thought, was an expertise that could analyze and make sense of the turmoil. I was wrong. My most valuable tool is words, the words I can now use only with difficulty. My voice is debilitated–mute, a prisoner of a communication system damaged by a stroke that has robbed me of language.

Individuals who have a stroke suffer a lone battle against the twin demons of frustration and depression. Their recovery period is maddeningly gradual. Some remain permanently incapacitated and unable to care for themselves. I am fortunate to have had sufficient recovery that I am physically independent; my ability to speak, however, is effortful and limited to short utterances.

Yet I keep forging ahead. Yes, it does take an ungodly amount of time. But I'll never stop trying. I have a strong desire to come out on top. Having the support of family and friends is essential. Anyone in this

---

Abraham H. Raskin served for many years as Deputy Director of the Editorial Page for *The New York Times*, and was the recipient of many prestigious awards in journalism. We regret that Mr. Raskin died shortly after having written this article.

Reprinted with permission of *Martha's Vineyard Magazine*, (Fall/Holiday, 1992).

[Haworth co-indexing entry note]: "The Words I Lost." Raskin, Abraham H. Co-published simultaneously in *Loss, Grief & Care* (The Haworth Press, Inc.) Vol. 8, No. 1/2, 1998, pp. 165-174; and: *After Stroke: Enhancing Quality of Life* (ed: Wallace Sife) The Haworth Press, Inc., 1998, pp. 165-174.

situation needs much love to get through this hell. Consider yourself lucky if your caring and understanding could bring success closer for those who have had a stroke and have suffered in silence.

The stroke happened in the Indian summer of September, 1990, a time of excitement, freedom and fun, when I truly experienced joie de vivre. I took delight in my good health and vigor as a widower of 80 years young. I had recently met Margorie Neikrug, curator of a photographic gallery and the woman who would later become my wife.

On September 29, a Saturday, Marge and I went to the funeral of a union leader at St. Patrick's Cathedral in Manhattan. We walked home and had lunch. Our plan was to catch a two o'clock train for Spring Valley to visit Marge's daughter. We never took the train.

During our lunch I noticed my right arm getting heavier and heavier, then I passed out. Marge realized I was in trouble and pushed me back into my chair. It took all her strength. Immediately she called 911 and also the men downstairs. The ambulance and the doormen arrived simultaneously.

The ambulance took me to the emergency room of New York Hospital, just a few blocks from home. There an experimental drug, Eminase, was recommended to prevent further damage.

But Eminase can be administered only with the consent of a blood relative. Marge, the closest person to me, could not provide that consent. Yet the drug must be given within three hours after the onset of the stroke to be effective. The next two hours were critical in determining my fate.

It was urgent for Marge to get a family member's consent on a sunny Saturday afternoon in September. Hysterically, she called the entire family, from California and Texas to New York, without success. "I was desperate," she said later. Time was running out. Finally my daughter-in-law, Linda, saved the day. She found my daughter, Jane, who gave consent. I received the medicine within the prescribed time.

The medical care was marvelous, with doctors and nurses in constant attendance. But for that team, I would not be here today. The CAT scan confirmed that I had suffered a cerebral vascular accident–in layman's terms, a stroke caused by an embolism (clot) blocking the blood flow to the main artery feeding the brain.

Unfortunately the team could not reverse the damage done to certain areas of my brain during the stroke. The site of the damage was within the left brain hemisphere in an area that controls speech, reading, comprehension and writing. The medical term for this disorder is aphasia. An estimated one million Americas suffer it.

I was a beaten-up character, shellshocked, disoriented and dazed, unaware of what was happening to me. I desperately wanted to make sense of the confusion, but every time I tried to express myself nothing came out. I was forced to remain silent and could not follow either verbal or written commands. Words sounded to me like jargon, as though the people around me spoke a foreign tongue. I could neither comprehend nor use verbal language. In addition, the stroke left my right arm and leg semi-paralyzed, thwarting my ability get up and walk independently. I lay in bed, staring blankly and feeling helpless.

Over the next few days, however, the doctors recorded marked improvement in my strength. The most notable and rapid accomplishment was to walk without any assistance. After long and tedious hours spent with Marge, where she rotated my legs and, most importantly, provided me with encouragement, it was a blessing to be able to walk to her once again.

My next feat occurred when I was able to lift my right arm up in the air above my head. Only constant effort by the nurses and technicians motivated me to continue trying. Each day I raised the arm to higher levels until finally reaching straight up. I felt like an eager schoolboy raising my hand to show the teacher that I was an A+ scholar.

Simultaneously my understanding of simple conversation was returning. With the steady acceleration in comprehension skills, the doctors tracked my ability to follow directions of increasing difficulty until I demonstrated that I was able to follow complex multi-level commands. In addition, I began to produce what I thought were words, but the puzzled look on the faces of the hearers showed me that my long-awaited words were nothing more than gibberish.

Then, little by little, people began reacting to my vocalizations, indicating that I was beginning to produce meaningful words. Imagine the relief at again being able to express my basic needs with a single word like "eat," "drink" or "toilet." Each utterance involved deep concentration and struggle to produce a somewhat intelligible word. Fortunately each "new" word was received with praise and elation by my family and friends, motivating me to go on. A baby must be excited like that when he utters his first "mama" and "dada."

The physical skills seemed to be coming back. There was some strength in my fingers on the right hand, although I was still not able to do tasks requiring fine motor coordination, such as writing, zippering and tying my shoes. In general, my partial paralysis improved and the affected limbs were functional, although the speed and precision of the movements was diminished.

The positive changes in my body encouraged me to believe that, with treatment, my communication skills would also improve. Therefore I applied immediately to the Rusk Institute of Rehabilitation Medicine for intense help in speech remediation.

"To believe in rehabilitation is to believe in humanity." Dr. Howard A. Rusk, the founder of the Institute of Rehabilitation Medicine, put forth his therapeutic philosophy to treat the whole man to solve, not only his physical but his emotional, social and psychological problems. His successors have followed Dr. Rusk's tradition and the institute has become one of the world's premier rehabilitation centers.

From my perspective, entering Rusk would guarantee a complete and rapid recovery. I commenced the program feeling optimistic and enthusiastic, eager to begin the regimen of daily drills including physical, occupational and speech therapy. Like a soldier ready for battle, I geared myself for combat against the enemy that had invaded my body. I was willing to do whatever was necessary to end this chapter of my life. My greatest wish was to return to my career as soon as possible.

Dr. Rusk's book, *A World To Care For*, was a tribute to the extraordinary achievements of thousands of disabled. With the proper training and understanding, they have overcome incredible physical disadvantages to become outstanding workers, citizens and members of their communities. These people–the quadriplegics, the paraplegics, the amputees and the like–are not complaining about their plights. If they could do it, then why couldn't I?

The support and guidance that I received from the professional staff was super. For instance, the occupational therapists focused upon fine motor movements in my right hand that would enable me to perform daily tasks such as using utensils, buttoning my clothing and holding a pen and pencil. At first, I had limited movement in my right arm. My right hand, in fact, was almost useless. My muscles were flaccid. The occupational therapists prodded me to expand upon whatever strength I could muster in my limp fingers. A lack of movement could result in a contracture producing deformity. Therefore I was presented with the most sophisticated equipment available to do the job. I never imagined that would mean putting pegs in slots, squeezing mesh pot scrubbers, stringing beads on a cord and pinching clothes-pins on horizontal bars. The fine motor movements that were damaged in my fingers made picking up small objects, using a fork or spoon, zippering my jacket or even inserting a key in a lock difficult to perform. Each week brought noticeable improvement in my dexterity.

While rehabilitating my hand, the therapist also worked on my weak facial muscles. The stroke had left me with a droop on the right side of my face. If this was purely cosmetic, I would not have been concerned. However, this muscle weakness made the right half of my mouth and tongue unable to hold back my saliva. The result was an endless cascade of drivel streaming out over my cheeks and chest, for which I had to carry a constant supply of wipes. The facial exercises consisted mainly of stretching in horrible contorted shapes, blowing bubbles, inflating balloons and moving a ball in mid-air by puffing through a pipe or straw. All of these exercises were in preparation for drinking from a cup without leakage. After many hours and many wet towels, I somehow managed to achieve this goal, though the drool still persists.

Of course, even Rusk was not heaven, and my zeal for progress sometimes bumped into the inevitable shortcomings of any bureaucracy. For instance, the fourth day Marge asked me when I had taken a shower. My reply, in sign language, was zero. Marge couldn't believe it. She raised hell and said she would not leave the hospital until I had been cleaned. Their curt answer: "We are out of towels." There was a three-hour delay before the towels arrived–at which time the orderlies were too busy to help me! We decided to break the rules and go it on our own. Marge escorted me into the shower room.

The next morning the orderlies again didn't know I needed attention: They had bathed the old patients and continued to ignore me. So I planned a strategy to evade the requirement that patients be escorted to the showers. At 6 AM each morning, with the side rails on the bed still up I would slither down to the side of the bed without being noticed. No one saw me get out of bed, so without assistance I went to the shower and washed. This was my clandestine scheme the rest of my stay at Rusk.

There were other bureaucratic issues at Rusk. Though I had entered Rusk fully ambulatory, the nurses insisted that I confine myself to a wheelchair. As a believer in passive resistance, I decided go on strike until they allowed me to walk on my own. I sat belligerently at the edge of my bed refusing to be carted in a wheelchair. For some hours the nurses were inflexible. Then they reluctantly investigated my complaint until finally receiving approval from the physical therapists to give in. After physical therapy workouts, I was rapidly dismissed. According to the therapists, I had demonstrated sufficient agility and strength in order to perform basic daily movements.

But the speech therapy, which I continued on a daily basis as an out-patient, was a laborious and disturbing battle. There was the worry about the outcome: Words had been the sustenance and the pleasure of my life, but now it was words that were letting me down. My body was nearly back to normal, but I felt that a black hole was swallowing my speech. Would it be realistic of me to assume that the complete physical recuperation would lead to a total reemergence of my language skills? Would all of this daily grind pay off? I persisted nonetheless, and the therapists pushed me to do more. For me, the aphasic patient, speech therapy would be my passport to humanity. The experience would never be forgotten. Helen Wulf once said she could "still feel the indescribable relief when a rescuing speech therapist opened the door. There was a golden thread linking us. It was my lifeline to sanity."

Home was the right place for me after a ten-day stay at Rusk. My great faith in recovery was tied to the warmth and encouragement of the domestic spirit. I constantly pushed myself forward, thriving on each modest improvement. I recognized the role of the outpatient: the struggle for independence.

My daily adventure from home started by taxi to 34th Street. Marge took me, screaming, "You can't go by yourself." Carmen, my practical nurse, usually called for me–until one fateful day she forgot. Pandemonium! Marge, Robyn, her granddaughter, and John Staszyn, the designer, were busy hanging a show at the gallery. Marge, white-faced, was startled to find that I had vanished. Cabs were taken to Rusk, to the police station, to home, to the gallery. Still no Abe.

About an hour later I walked in nonchalantly on my own steam. I had no choice. I didn't carry any money for a phone call or for bus fare. I decided that from that day forward I was on my own. After that my legs became my main source of transportation. I walked almost all of the time, except during the rain and snow when I allowed myself the luxury of a bus or taxi. The one-hour hike, to and fro, was a 35-block commute each way.

At Rusk, my primary goal in therapy was to recapture the words that would no longer roll off the tip of my tongue as trippingly as they once did. I was now an aphasic, a person who suffered difficulty in communication as a result of the brain damage incurred during my stroke. Before this incident, I had never heard of the term "aphasia." Now I learned first hand all the psychosocial consequences that came from an inability to speak. I felt psychologically isolated.

It is difficult to convey the depth of my emotional solitude. I did not feel like A. H. Raskin. I now had a new "self," a person who no longer could use words with the mastery that led me to receive awards and medals annually. The finest tribute came from the men at the copy desk. "Reading Abe's copy is like ice cream," they said. Now, it may take as much as an hour to formulate a single written sentence. I know exactly what I want to express, but transferring the words to paper is a rigorous job. I persist, nonetheless. I am resolute to overcome my handicap.

Martha Taylor Sarno, president of the National Aphasia Association, who is also the director of the Rusk Speech Department, wrote a simple little book called *Understanding Aphasia*, which explains in plain words the nature of the affliction and how much could be done to overcome it. "Aphasia is a nightmare of a disorder," says Dr. Sarno. "To have language taken away is far worse than any other loss a person could sustain." One of the reasons is that aphasia does not resemble a physical disability. The public knows how to respond to someone who uses a wheelchair or who walks with crutches. Aphasia, however, has no physical signs. One mild aphasic whose physical disabilities had been resolved said, "I wish my arm were open and bleeding so that people could see that something is wrong." Aphasia remains a mystery to the general population. As the National Aphasia Association survey concluded: "Many people don't even know the word aphasia, much less what it does to you."

The social isolation resulting from difficulty in communication has a profound impact on the aphasic person and his family. Feelings range from frustration, depression, grief and anger to passivity and helplessness. Aphasics are often compelled to withdraw during social situations, feeling like an "outsider" in their own home. It's a very lonely life.

Privately I could do nothing but cry. With the tears came feelings of anxiety and depression. I wondered if the emptiness would ever go away. I wavered back and forth between feelings of melancholy and those of hope. I always knew how fortunate I was to have family and friends in my life, who provided endless love and support. My children Jane and Don and my brother Bernie were always by my side. Whether through long distance phone calls or in weekly visits, they always expressed their love and devotion. Marge, a mainstay of inspiration and faith, has provided me with ongoing encouragement, cheerleading for me all the while.

The desire to achieve, to succeed, to win, to regain my confidence manifested itself in the practice that Marge and I incorporated into our daily routine. Every night I challenged Marge to a game. It became our happy hour. We played, joked and enjoyed the frolic. Whether it's dominoes, bingo or backgammon, the one invariable rule is that Marge can't win and I can't lose. I'm such a sorehead.

I approached this problem with all my might. I attended Rusk daily for both individual and group speech therapy. Debra Wiener, cheerful and with a keen mind, was the head of the expert team. Activities presented ranged from speech stimulation to use of the computer. Long hours were spent relearning the basics–counting, ABCs, the days of the week, simple conversation. In the beginning I carried a pocket notebook containing lists of words describing emotions, family names, days, objects, foods, etc. If a word did not come, I could refer to my notebook for assistance.

The speech clarity was poor because of weak facial muscles so I had to focus on improving my articulation skills. I sat before a mirror with Debbie, intently studying each movement of her mouth and trying to imitate her with as much accuracy as possible. I was drilled to respond to word retrieval tasks such as finding opposites, sentence production, and sentence formulation. Simultaneously we worked upon my reading, writing and spelling, which had also been affected by my stroke. I practiced on the computer, searching for errors in spelling, grammar and syntax.

In spite of the slow but steady progress that I achieved in speech therapy, I found myself feeling awkward and self-conscious during social situations. Whether in aphasia class or at home with friends, I groped for the words but they didn't come. I became bashful and morose. People allowed me the time to express myself, but I gave up. It was like not being able to say an old friend's name, multiplied to infinity.

As preparations were under way for our annual pilgrimage to Martha's Vineyard, Marge made arrangements for a therapist to work with me at our home on the Island. Donna Rhoades of the Vineyard Nursing Association was a buoyant and upbeat therapist who drilled me day in and day out during our four-month stay.

The enticement of the natural Island beauty—its beaches, sparkling ocean, brilliant sunshine and the merriment of the vacationers—was temptation enough for me to chuck my notebooks. Donna, my coach, inspired me to keep plugging away, however. We worked as a team. Collaborating with Donna was stimulating. She presented me with a steady supply of materials aimed at helping me to combine spoken words automatically, to produce simple sentences and later to begin to formulate questions. We worked endlessly on numbers, but to this day that remains my nemesis.

The progress I made that summer restored my confidence and my drive to keep on trying. On my return to New York I was full of pep, joy and enthusiasm. I commenced therapy with Randi Jacoby, a private speech pathologist who came well-recommended. She works with me one hour daily, in contrast to my former half-hour at Rusk. I have been able to speed up my progress with this charming, chatty pathologist. She has a radiance about her person. She is skillful in handling my shyness, inventive and intelligent in her treatment. I am lucky to have her.

The skilled speech therapist, Dr. Sarno has said, is constantly balancing linguistic recovery factors against human needs. "The effective therapist is a forgiving, accepting and approving patient ally. While functioning as an advocate, she must be completely knowledgeable about the details of what the patient can and cannot do." I am fortunate that my three thera-pists have all responded to me in this way.

Reading was my next problem area. The printed word initially re-sembled hieroglyphics. Later, individual words became recognizable and took on meaning, but I could not decipher a printed statement. Looking at a group of words was overwhelming. It was as though the words were catapulting off the page and could not make sense of their significance. It was grueling to pick up a newspaper. How depressed I felt when I couldn't read *The New York Times*, my lifeline for over 50 years. The therapist presented two words, three words, four words and more until I graduated to sentences. Randi and I took apart individual headlines and sentences from the daily edition of *The Times* until I mastered reading an article as a whole.

What pained me more than anything was being a writer who could no longer write. I felt dismembered. After the stroke I was left not only without speech, but without the ability to spell a simple word. At first I felt mournful and frightened, then tense, anxious and full of rage. Yet I knew that I had to get back on that horse.

Initially, when I tried to write my name, I just scribbled. Slowly, by copying the letters over and over, it began to come back to me. Spelling was no longer automatic. I was drilled to put down letters and words to dictation, finish the spelling of incomplete words and look for errors in misspelled words. Gradually I combined words in order to form sentences, although I tended to omit the articles and prepositions. Verb tense was yet another chore. I had to rethink all of the irregular and plural forms before printing it out.

Through all the darkness, my guiding light was and always will be my dear Marge. Blithe in spirit, witty and wistful, she was my live-in love. I saw a new side of her after my accident. I thought of her as a valiant saint forging on to save the lives of snowbound travelers in the St. Bernard Pass. She was my angel of mercy, unselfish, gentle, kind, loyal and always sympathetic.

With a mutual feeling of commitment, we were married on December 5, 1990. The consecration of our love deepened through concern, devo-tion and tenderness. It gave us great joy to have family and friends join us on our double celebration in a reaffirmation of our vows at the National Arts Club on my 80th birthday. I wrote a poem, which I was unable to read. The Rabbi tenderly recited each word for me:

I thank my beautiful bride.
I marvel at your strength,

caring and charm.
You have been at my side
Through the greatest battle
of my life.
And because of you,
I am winning that battle.
I love you, Marge.

I now realize that my vocation in life has changed. I have and always will be the "voice of the people." But now I represent the one million Americans who cannot speak for themselves. My plight and theirs are one: to inform the public that those of us who have lost the ability to invent phrases or sentences in a fluent manner have not lost the ability to think. We retain the skill to communicate our thoughts and feelings, whether through writing, picture boards, pantomime or facial expression. We can still speak! We hope that you will listen with your ears, with your eyes and always with your heart.

Aphasia,
as Seen by an Aphasic

Hermine Koplin Kutscher

It is extremely difficult for an aphasic person to communicate what he or she thinks or feels, and what it is like, suffering from that disability. This essay took Hermine Koplin Kutscher about two and a half months to put together. Under normal circumstances she probably could have written it in about an hour. Despite her frustrating handicap, she worked very hard describing this personal experience. In reading it we get an intimate perspective of what it is like to be aphasic. This also offers us some inspirational insight into the personal drive and dynamism of a woman who would not succumb to the ravages of stroke. (Austin H. Kutscher)

Aphasia means a lonely existence. Your mind works all the time. You become exhausted from trying to tell people what you are thinking. I find that when I am tired or excited, it is better to keep quiet instead of saying things that are incorrect or irrelevant. That is a lonely existence. I was very active and articulate before I had a stroke, which was in August 1991. I had lost my 13 year old dog, Trumpet, in July of that year. She was more than a pet. She had been a champion in dog shows. She was a therapy dog, and we had visited schools, hospitals, nursing homes and institutions for the handicapped. In my home, she would greet family

Hermine Koplin Kutscher authored numerous articles and books on pets, and was one of the founders of the Pet Therapy Movement, devoting much of her time taking therapy dogs on visits to nursing homes. We deeply regret that Mrs. Kutscher died in 1996.

[Haworth co-indexing entry note]: "Aphasia, as Seen by an Aphasic." Kutscher, Hermine Koplin. Co-published simultaneously in *Loss, Grief & Care* (The Haworth Press, Inc.) Vol. 8, No. 1/2, 1998, pp. 175-177; and: *After Stroke: Enhancing Quality of Life* (ed: Wallace Sife) The Haworth Press, Inc., 1998, pp. 175-177. Single or multiple copies of this article are available for a fee from The Haworth Document Delivery Service [1-800-342-9678, 9:00 a.m. - 5:00 p.m. (EST). E-mail address: getinfo@haworth.com].

and visitors by jumping on them. Yet, she would never jump on an individual, if sick or disabled.

Once when visiting a hospital, a man signaled that he wanted to touch her. I didn't know at the time that he was nonverbal. When it was time for Trumpet and me to leave, the man helped me gather our belongings and uttered the words, "I love that dog." Those were apparently his first words. He had aphasia and couldn't talk. Now, I know what's it's like, a lonely existence!

Trumpet was slowing down in her last two years. I took her to the Animal Medical Center where she had four acupuncture treatments for arthritis. She responded like a young dog and was good for a year. But, then she had strokes. First, my dog, then me. It was eerie.

My stroke evolved over a week period of time. I didn't know I was having a stroke. I was told that I was having a nervous breakdown. I knew something was wrong and was glad someone had pinpointed the problem. I accepted it since I had so recently lost Trumpet. I recall vacationing in the Poconos, and my sister had come to visit. I was saying something about "Bear's coming" and it was irrelevant. I was laughing excessively. My sister noticed, but it soon went away.

I really don't remember how it came to be that I was hospitalized. My neurologist reported possible changes in my right hand. I was then sent for various tests and my symptoms worsened. I couldn't talk or use my right hand or leg. I received therapy as an inpatient for seven weeks, and then continued as an outpatient. The first year, I made the most progress, however.

I am still going for speech therapy and do not want to stop. I want to continue to improve my speech and need the stimulation and support I receive in therapy. I have worked on finding strategies to help me get my words out. It's exhausting and frustrating at times. I'm now able to carry on short conversations, but I depend on having a good and patient listener as I struggle along. Not everyone fits the bill, and that contributes to my loneliness.

I avoid using the telephone, unless necessary. I don't often travel alone, even though I drive again. I carry a card with me that says I have trouble speaking. My life has changed in other ways. My endurance is not what it used to be and I have had to make adjustments. I need to sit down frequently. My shopping trips are short. I take someone with me because I cannot carry packages. I buy more from catalogs now. I have been fortunate enough to drive again, however, I stick to the side streets and take short trips. It takes a lot of energy and concentration to drive and I tire quickly.

I have had to learn to use my left hand as my dominant hand. Though I have movement in my right arm and hand, I don't have the strength. I am not able to keep up the household and so I have hired help. I can do laundry but can't carry it up the stairs. I can no longer mend my clothing. I have two dogs that require care and I need assistance in preparing their food.

My social life has been significantly changed. I was extremely active before the stroke, particularly in my work with my therapy dog, Trumpet, as well as with dog shows. I lectured and wrote articles and a book. My husband's work also involves many symposiums, dinners and ceremonies, in which I actively participated. I can no longer take part in most of these activities as I don't have the stamina, nor do I have the communication skills needed. I have found that, regardless of people's concern about my well being, most are uncomfortable with the changes I am faced with. It takes some skills to learn to communicate effectively with an aphasic individual. And, most people are unfortunately either unwilling or unable to develop that skill. That, too, is why aphasia means a lonely existence.

EDITOR NOTE

Hermine Koplin Kutscher died from lung cancer after this was written. She was a remarkable woman, who fought very hard every day of her life to overcome the ravages of her stroke. This essay is only part of the legacy of hope and smiles she has left us. Despite her disability she worked relentlessly to regain the quality of life she wanted, and offers inspiration to us all, by this living example.

Wallace Sife

The Language Loss
of Patricia Neal and Helen Wulf

Barbara Newborn

In searching for literature that offers a personal account of stroke and resultant loss of language, the personal experiences of Patricia Neal and Helen Wulf are outstanding.[1,2] They both portray keen insight into the aphasic experience. From this we can more clearly understand where the communication breakdown occurs, and learn to appreciate its importance in our relationships with ourselves and others.

PATRICIA NEAL

Patricia Neal suffered her stroke February 17, 1965. She was pregnant, and at home when she lost consciousness. After 22 days of silence, she finally uttered a word, but nothing came after it. Prior to that she had been an award-winning actress. Now her articulation was slow, and too easily misperceived as a drunken slur, although she didn't have as monotonous a way of talking as other aphasics. The limits of her vocabulary were made evident through her speech, which was punctuated with formulas and spacefillers. Formulaic speech would give her a false sense of security. She also had word blockage of the very familiar names in her life. They could be of a past director, a movie she played in, or even a character she had portrayed.

Barbara Newborn is Chief of Staff and National Spokesperson for the NSEI, and has just completed a book based upon her personal experiences with stroke.

[Haworth co-indexing entry note]: "The Language Loss of Patricia Neal and Helen Wulf." Newborn, Barbara. Co-published simultaneously in *Loss, Grief & Care* (The Haworth Press, Inc.) Vol. 8, No. 1/2, 1998, pp. 179-187; and: *After Stroke: Enhancing Quality of Life* (ed: Wallace Sife) The Haworth Press, Inc., 1998, pp. 179-187. Single or multiple copies of this article are available for a fee from The Haworth Document Delivery Service [1-800-342-9678, 9:00 a.m. - 5:00 p.m. (EST). E-mail address: getinfo@haworth.com].

She went blank when she tried to think of names. Sometimes the best she could do was come up with a nonsense word that sounded like the word she wanted to remember. Her deficits in memory led her to believe her acting ability was gone. She tried to ascribe this new difficulty to poor eyesight and not her mind.

Her reading and speaking ability was impaired, and she read aloud very slowly, with poor articulation. She had a monotonous tone, whether relating a story, joke, or even a prayer. She had difficulty remembering many words, and suffered a general loss of comprehension, as well as poor retention. She also displayed poor recall of spelling and had difficulty with certain sentence formations.

At extreme moments, Pat felt that she was going crazy. She said to her husband, Roald, that she hadn't had a dream since her stroke. Like many others, she mistakenly linked her speechlessness, dreamlessness, and the like with insanity. It was hard to see herself as normal. She felt too different. What kind of self-image could she have had when she couldn't even remember the months of the year?

At first Neal didn't understand one word that she read. She and her husband tried to read Hemingway because of the short, plain sentences, but the ideas were still too complex for her.

Roald set her up with strenuous speech and physical therapy exercises. She didn't mind the speech therapy. In fact, she looked forward to it. There was tremendous excitement in working with the therapist, as she progressed every day. She even looked for her teacher's car and waited for him to come and start the lessons so that she could relearn more. She wanted the words and their meanings pulled out of her brain, where they would begin to open up a whole new world. She wanted to understand life again, but first there was so much more to uncover in her mind.

Pat tried reading *Peter Rabbit* to her son. She read it in a flat uncomprehending voice, studying each word with hard concentration, putting the stresses in the wrong places. Pat began to hate these little rodents with their uncomprehended lines that reminded her of her failures. Finally, she threw down the book in exasperation. She didn't understand what she was trying to read.

Writing was a relief and comfort for her, and the only way she could communicate fully. She found this the best way to express her thoughts, and was amazed with all the things that she remembered in her compositions. She could not believe how much of her past she remembered, and wrote of the past lives of her grandfather and her father, as well as the type of life she had led.

Pat would send tapes to her friends instead of writing letters. Her tapes were two minutes long, but it took her over an hour to get the words right. She wanted them to be perfect, but often she would just draw a blank and forget what she wanted to say. Finally she used cue cards, even though her reading was poor. She sometimes had to re-record at least twelve times before getting an acceptable take.

Singing songs helped her with word meanings. Pat remembered and practiced songs she had known twenty years before. The words all did come back, and Pat joined Roald in singing them. Pat's singing demonstrated that her voice was not impaired. Her voice had always been the most distinctive quality of her acting, especially since she could use it to give a hundred different effects.

Seeing many of her supportive friends again boosted her spirits. Her closest friend, Anne Bancroft, was sensitive enough to know when to speak and when not to, thus allowing Pat to utter the few words she knew. However, other visitors seemed at their wits' ends after five minutes with her. It required considerable perception to decide whether Pat's lagging conversation was due to speechlessness or simple mindedness. Those who guessed speechlessness talked incessantly during their visits. Others thought Pat had regressed to childhood, and condescendingly spoke to her in baby talk.

Pat was confused about her intelligence. This was made a greater problem when some visitors wrongly assumed that intelligence also was always demonstrated by one's speaking ability. While receiving company, Pat hardly spoke more than one word, if there were more than one person in the room. It was hard for her to deal with the fast rate of conversations. So she either remained silent or did all the talking.

Pat's impairments not only frustrated her when company was in the room, but also while watching TV. Her eyes were glued to the set, on the night of the Oscar awards. When Audrey Hepburn said, "We're all pulling for Pat Neal who couldn't be here tonight," Pat felt cheated that she couldn't be there, sharing in all the glamour. She feared that the world would soon forget her, because of the stroke.

She had moments of joy with her children, and these kept up her perseverance. One of the delights in Pat's life was Theo, her hydrocephalic child. He was an inspiration to her, as he too, had brain damage, and was overcoming it. His appearance made her realize the miracle of recovery. His mother's appearance and her silence puzzled Theo, but it gave him a chance to talk. He would visit her, aping the speech therapist's methods in teaching Pat how to read, write, and speak again. When the therapist left, Theo brought Pat his flash cards and checked her on words he knew.

Pat began to feel that her willful personality would help make everything all right, again. She had the hope to be her old self again, but it required courage to take certain risks. Three months after her stroke, May 17, she flew to Washington, D.C., and spent the day with the Kennedys. Her spirits were cheerful and she was more talkative than she had been in California. The whole day was a success in her eyes, and she provided delightful company for the president and his wife.

Her second risk was her public appearance in a press conference when she was leaving the U.S. to go to London. The conference was successful and, that return to the public eye bolstered and encouraged her. Responses from people in each of these settings gave her the kind of support she needed. Pat knew that to become the person she was before, she needed to push herself to the limit. However, each new social situation had its own elements of risk.

Clearly, it was the support Pat Neal received that made it possible for her to return to her former life. Positive feedback from friends was very encouraging. She was amazed when those who hadn't seen her for a few months, raved about her progress. She also received and answered many letters from other stroke survivors. Patricia Neal became an important public figure, who inspired courage.

The next big risk was when she was the main speaker at the Waldorf, in New York, in a program for the benefit of brain damaged people. In order to recover her presence on stage, she needed to push herself into overcoming her fears of speaking in public. She exerted much will to do this. Pat recognized the importance of social interaction to recovery, and the support of her audience pulled her through. When she stood up at the podium the crowd gave her a standing ovation. The speech had been taped, and later she listened to it, over and over again.

After six months, Pat's vanity began to return. She began to wear lipstick, and asked everyone how she looked. Her children were more comfortable with her, and she could put them to bed as she used to, read them a story, and tuck them in. Her friends responded to her improved speech and appearance with the feedback she needed. About a month after the baby's birth, things began to improve, steadily.

Pat's friends held a dinner, honoring her. They drank many toasts, and praised her for her strength and capacity for life. The dinner seemed to mark an end to the deepest worries for her future—indeed, it was true that things were returning to normal. Though Pat was still apologetic and sometimes depressed, she talked and laughed like a person with hopes for the future. Even the major accomplishments Pat could claim were not sufficient.

When she was about 80 percent recovered, Pat believed she would not improve any more. She wanted to sit back and do nothing, but Roald kept pushing her into strenuous therapy and visits to neighbors. Her next stage of improvement came when she began to joke with strangers. And Pat began to realize that people still loved her.

In due time, she was sent to Washington to receive from President Johnson the American Heart Association Award. On the flight, the plane started having mechanical difficulties. She even tried making the other passengers feel better, getting their minds off the problem by asking them questions, such as how many children they had.

Pat's final sense of restored identity came from making the picture, *The Subject Was Roses*. When she started filming, her commitment was strong. But at the beginning, she was terribly afraid of not knowing her lines, and had several disappointments.

She was constantly afraid of giving a bad performance. She also was terribly anxious about her first acting job, following the stroke since it would show what she was really capable of. The public would be watching her carefully and critically because they knew about her come-back from aphasia. She was not at all sure that she wanted to be in the public eye again.

She had to work diligently against her anxieties, which made it hard to use language. She feared that she had lost her acting ability, and wondered how could she act when her aphasia left her without the ability to memorize lines. The lines were mostly short, but Pat still had trouble learning them. She thought that the crew would have to coach her with all sorts of cue cards. And even with their help she would probably forget.

Pat was miserable after a only one week of rehearsing for the film. She had to go over the same scene 26 times. Never before had this happened to her. Instead of saying the lines right, she would say the wrong word in trial after trial, or she would use her formulaic speech, or she would keep silent. The 27th time, Pat finally said the lines correctly, and laughed. But the newspaper headlines made her a heroine. At first, she neither understood nor spoke about this.

By the time the picture was finished, her healing was complete. When Pat saw the previews of the film, she was finally able to confirm her recovery to herself. The night of the premiere she was in her glory, surrounded by photographers. The persuasive force of friends and the ability to view completed work had been major factors in her recovery. Patricia Neal regained her acting skill and became again the dedicated and disciplined actress that she had been.

HELEN WULF

Helen Wulf suffered a stroke February 3, 1970. She was middle-aged at the time. For about twenty years prior to the stroke she was associated with her husband in his business, as a sales representative for children's apparel manufacturers.

At the time of the stroke, she did not know what was happening to her. She was completely unaware of her language loss, and that she could not comprehend the gravity of the situation. She even thought it strange that her husband should call her son to come right down. She appeared to become more unaware as the day went on, and became increasingly oblivious and euphoric.

Eventually, when her speech began to return, it was an exhausting process to find the right words, and then to say them. At first, her words were unintelligible. When she was fatigued she made more mistakes than usual. Helen compared her aphasic speaking to a short circuited computer because she felt she must find roundabout methods to improvise, using parts of the brain that were still in good shape. Speaking, to her, was always conscious and deliberate—and not automatic. It was an exhausting task. She had many thoughts, and they had to be put into inner speech before speaking out. But because it was a conscious and deliberate act, she was elated with even the smallest accomplishment.

At the hospital, two days after her stroke, Helen Wulf experienced her initial shock at not being able to communicate. When she was eager to share an experience with two nurses, a sudden sense of frustration overwhelmed her, because only jargon came out.

She had memory losses, and even could not remember the name of her speech problem. But she thought she understood what people were saying to her. The only way she could find words was to capture them in syllables. She brought the root to mind and then struggled with suffixes and prefixes. She reports frequent word blockage. Like other aphasics, as she began to get back words, she found herself limited and confused. She couldn't assimilate words properly because her internal and external vocabularies were in disrepair.

At the onset of her stroke, Wulf continually wondered if she was a vegetable. Because of the aphasic's inability to speak such doubts, they can become self-fulfilling prophecy. Many people misperceive the aphasic as mindless, and he can't help reacting to those callous comments. Because of the aphasic's inability to speak he may feel, as Wulf did, hopeless and helpless as a baby. Wulf couldn't tell others that she had to go to the bathroom. She couldn't stop crying when her minister entered the hospital room. She didn't understand what he was doing there and what he was saying. She wanted to respond to him, but she couldn't speak. She couldn't question her husband, Hans, to find out what was wrong with her. All these experiences forced a great sense of helplessness on her.

She needed people who could talk to her, and understand her struggle. Wulf related well to her family and her speech therapist, but she was anxious outside of her private world. She saw that society could not understand or put up with her errors, and that embarrassed and upset her.

Helen Wulf constantly mispronounced words, and felt her brain didn't sort words fast enough or put them in their proper order. Her tongue got tied up, making it hard to pronounce polysyllabic words. When she tried to speak such words, it was as if each sound were a single word, in itself. Her laughter was also distorted because of her poor articulation. It became an uncontrollable, noisy, loud spurt. Her singing voice was strangely pitched and off-key. It sounded to her like screeching. Her oral reading was monotonous and done in a breathless, shaky voice.

Impaired vocabulary recall required mental acrobatics to find a word or a synonym. At those times it took considerable effort for her not to lose her train of thought. Sometimes her vocabulary would not come to mind at all, and for that moment the thought was lost. This sometimes resulted in her using words she never intended.

If she didn't write her thoughts down they would quickly be forgotten. To write she often had to look up the spelling of every word, even though she couldn't even remember the letter it started with. Helen had been a good speller before the stroke, but two years later, her spelling remained terrible.

Poor hand coordination interfered with her writing. Like most aphasics, she had to learn to write with the left hand. Because of that, writing during the first few weeks was a tremendous task. Each single sentence was a great accomplishment, since she had to overcome awkwardness in her hand, as well as her defective sentence formulation and poor recall. When Wulf returned from the hospital she knew that writing would be her best way of communicating. This activity also enabled her to think in abstractions, again. When that finally happened, her past, present and future suddenly returned to their proper prospectives.

As to reading impairments, the first time she looked at a newspaper, all the words were meaningless; they were a jumble of letters signifying nothing. Comprehending a short article took intense concentration. Before her stroke, Helen delighted in books and words. But afterward, even the cards and letters she received were difficult for her to understand. She remembered little of what she read, even from short passages. When she tried to read newspaper comics, she couldn't see any humor to them.

When listening, Wulf's major impairment was confusion, caused by noise. She reported that individual conversations could not be differentiated when there are several voices in a room. Because of this she misinterpreted words said to her. In the early days after the stroke she could not talk, and had disturbing thoughts from misinterpreting what other people said to her. For instance, while in the hospital she listened to her minister pray and felt disheartened because she misinterpreted his words and couldn't even remember them a moment later. Gradually, however, she regained her ability to listen to one conversation at a time–and could do so accurately, if she was not distracted.

In order to make progress in speech, Helen felt she had to continue to use her voice to find new pathways. She felt that the more she was involved in interpersonal communication, the more her speech would recover. She saw herself as a thinking human being though it was difficult for her to verbalize her thoughts to others.

Wulf noted that she had previously been able to sort out many conversations, as at a social affair. Social affairs once delighted her, but now they became a mass of confusion. Constant and rapid speech frustrated her. If a meeting involved more than six people, it turned into a cacophony of sounds. She could not sort out separate conversations.

Helen commented that she always had to think before speaking, and sounded as if she had an accent. Prior to aphasia she did not consciously think about every single phrase before speaking.

She recalled that she used to speak automatically and effortlessly, and now speech was a conscious and exhausting process. Another problem she perceived was her difficulty in making everyday decisions, like what to wear and what to cook. She reported having many thoughts, all competing at the same time.

In speaking, it was hard to find the right words and to remember them while consciously organizing sentences. The process was further complicated by anxiety about the possible negative responses a listener might get. To do all these activities at once was an exhausting process. Difficulties in internal speech affected her in other ways. Her speech muscles tired easily, and her tongue was uncoordinated. It twisted over syllables all the more, when she was fatigued.

She feared phone calls because of substitution and word blocks. When she couldn't avoid being on the telephone, Helen often drew a complete blank. When asked for her phone number, she often couldn't remember. Because the caller can't be seen, she often forgot whom she was speaking with, or what the call was about.

Other problems Wulf reported were connected with making decisions or giving directions. Even when she had her ideas in order, they would not come out that way. She states that correcting one error after the other was fatiguing and eventually, though she was aware of her errors, she gave up correcting them. Many times she wanted to say something, but found it impossible to speak because of fatigue. Often, when talking she had great thoughts, but no way of expressing them.

People may regard the aphasic as depressed because of his perceived condition. But for the most part, it was her inability to communicate that frustrated Helen. She reported that while at the hospital she had no control or words to express what she thought. The first evening, the doctor believed he had explained what had happened to her. But she misunderstood, thinking she had been told that there was no brain damage. Then she wondered why she had paralysis and aphasia. The doctor had just said that her mind was intact, but not the brain.

Helen Wulf eloquently reminds us that the aphasic is a person with intelligence and love, and strong feelings. But when one suddenly loses the ability to communicate, it is devastating. Like Patricia Neal, she saw that determination, courage, humor, and a positive self-image were vital for her recovery. And she lived to prove this.

REFERENCES

1. Farrell, B., *Pat and Roald*, NY: Random House, 1969.
2. Wulf, H., *Aphasia, My World Alone*, Detroit: Wayne State U. Press, 1973.

Self-Portrait of an Aphasic
(from a Personal and Professional
Viewpoint)

Barbara Newborn

On June 7, 1973, at the age of 21, I suffered a stroke leaving me hemiplegic and aphasic. Suddenly, I had lost my ability to think and express myself in words. I was unable to understand spoken or written language. This was a horror for me, especially since I had just graduated from Ithaca College, and was about to begin my career as a speech and English teacher.

My language loss devastated me. I had not known how important language was in my daily life, until I lost it. I felt alone, surrounded by darkness, cut off from the rest of the world, because I couldn't communicate. Even a two-year-old could speak better than I. I could not think in sentences or even symbols. I could only hold images in present time. It was as though my mind had been emptied of words.

There was no way to express my feelings or ideas. I could no longer persuade or influence, or delight in the sound of my voice. I could not make polite talk, ask simple questions, or even make requests. I was unable to count to ten, or tell stories as I used to. I felt my whole personality was gone. I thought no one would ever know Barbara Newborn, again, but me, and in time, I would forget, because I had no words to remind me who I was.

I could not live for the future because, for the first time in my life I was

---

Barbara Newborn is Chief of Staff and National Spokesperson for the NSEI, and has just completed a book based upon her personal experiences with stroke.

[Haworth co-indexing entry note]: "Self-Portrait of an Aphasic (from a Personal and Professional Viewpoint)." Newborn, Barbara. Co-published simultaneously in *Loss, Grief & Care* (The Haworth Press, Inc.) Vol. 8, No. 1/2, 1998, pp. 189-200; and: *After Stroke: Enhancing Quality of Life* (ed: Wallace Sife) The Haworth Press, Inc., 1998, pp. 189-200. Single or multiple copies of this article are available for a fee from The Haworth Document Delivery Service [1-800-342-9678, 9:00 a.m. - 5:00 p.m. (EST). E-mail address: getinfo@haworth.com].

189

afraid of the future and what it held for me. I did not know if I would ever be able to communicate again, or what I would be capable of in my new and future life. I could only try to live in the present. Every day I waited for that half-hour speech therapy lesson and wondered, "When, oh when, will I be 'normal,' be human and communicate like everybody else." Every inch of progress meant something. Saying one more word, reading to the end of a picture book or relating to my father on our morning walks were terribly important. I remember crying, becoming angry, and even sometimes slamming a door or throwing down objects, all because of feelings of frustration about not being able to relate to anyone but myself.

I have now regained about 85-90 percent of my language abilities. But I am still aware of problems because of the last 10-15 percent. I am aware of it when I have a lot to say, but others don't understand because my sentence structure is incorrect or my speech is slurred. When in a group discussion I have something important to say, but I can't express it quickly enough, and lose my chance. I feel it when I give street directions, and do not know where to start. Short, precise thoughts overload my mind with tension. While writing this essay I am particularly aware of my loss. I know the essence of what I want to say but often am not able to write it down.

Because of my experience in losing, and then slowly regaining my language, I puzzled about how other aphasics reacted to their communication loss. What do they say about their language impairment and how it affects them and their relationship with others? Do they experience the same problems of word choice, poor spelling and slurred speech?

I also feel that it is important to gain insight into what aphasics say about their problems, for they were, at one time, people who could talk without conscious effort, and then, suddenly, could not do so any more. If they were lucky, they gradually regained some of their former language abilities. But aphasics rarely recover completely.

These people are the only ones who can tell us what it feels like to be aphasic, and what it's like to have language and lose it. They can give us insights into the importance of communication, and begin to tell us where breakdowns of language occur, and where specific problems lie in the components of reading, writing, listening and speaking. When we study language through those who lost it, we can begin to understand fully and appreciate its importance in our relationships with ourselves, and others.

This essay deals with a study of perceptions and reports by and about persons who suffered aphasia, in each of the four language components:

- Listening
- Reading

- Speaking
- Writing

I investigated, further:

1. What are characteristics of impairment in each of the given components?
2. What are the effects of these impairments on the aphasic's behavior?
3. What are the effects of these impairments on the aphasic's relationships with others?

I searched for anything that could give me personal accounts of language loss, and located approximately thirty technical articles from journals dealing with communication and aphasia. They tended to agree that aphasia is a communication disorder which affects the whole being, and it is not only a physical problem, but a social and emotional one, as well.

It also became clear from this review of literature that there was little or nothing written from the standpoint of the aphasic's own answers to questions like: What are the feelings and experiences that the patient is going through during his language loss? What is it really like to lose, without any warning, the ability to speak? And does this language loss affect or filter the aphasiac's personality or his relationships? Most articles found in this search were scientific and technical. They reported experimental and case studies, therapy techniques, or were neurology reports on brain lesions of stroke patients.

At last I came upon literature that contained more extensive, personal accounts. I used these books exclusively, in this essay, to try to answer the above three questions:

- Barry Farrell, *Pat and Roald*, Random House, New York
- Eric Hodgins, *Episode*, Athenaeum, New York
- Carmen McBride, *Silent Victory*, Nelson Hall Company, Chicago
- Scott Moss, *Recovery with Aphasia*, University of Illinois Press, Chicago
- Helen Wulf, *My World Alone*, Wayne State University Press, Detroit

Joseph Keenan's book, *A Procedure Manual in Speech Pathology with Brain-Damaged Adults*[1] (not listed above) states that aphasia is a linguistic loss which crosses over the linguistic components of reading, writing, listening and speaking. I used Keenan's classification system, which best explains impaired behaviors in these components. Following, is a brief summary of that system.

I. IMPAIRMENTS OF LISTENING

Shortened Auditory Retention Span. Some aphasics can not listen to long and complex instructions or repeat words or phrases.

Defective Speech Recognition and Interpretation. Some aphasics react as if a speaker were using jargon or nonsense words, or even mumbling phrases. This class of impairments also includes the inability to discriminate between different words. For example, you might ask an aphasic how he is today, and his reply might be his age. This is commonly called "word deafness" or "agnosia."

Slow Reaction Time. This means exactly what it states. Some aphasics, while listening, will not understand a statement if the speaking rate is rapid or even normal, or if the rhythm is off.

II. IMPAIRMENTS OF SPEAKING

Motor Speech Difficulty (Articulation). Some aphasics have certain vocal muscles paralyzed (i.e., lips, palates, larynx, or tongue). As a result, when they speak, they lose precision, and articulation comes out as slurred speech. Some aphasics sound as though they were drunk. This is called dysarthric speech. I use the expression "some aphasics" because aphasics have extremely varying degrees of impairment.

Impaired Vocabulary (Recall). This is known as anomia or word-finding difficulty. This inability to provide words produces long pauses, delayed responses, slow and hesitant rate of speech, and sound substitution. It is a semantic problem.

Nonsense Words or Jargon. Some aphasics' vocabularies are made up of meaningless words which are unintelligible to listeners, but may not be to the aphasic. The aphasic's speech may sound like a foreign language, or even gibberish.

Defective Sentence Formulation. Some aphasics find the words they want to use, but don't know how to organize them into sentences. This implies a difficulty with syntax, and is also characterized by a slow and hesitant rate of speech.

III. IMPAIRMENTS OF READING

Impaired Visual Recognition. Some aphasics may have impaired visual fields: a loss of vision. This interferes with reading because the aphasic may only see part of the page, paragraph or sentence. But he can compensate for this defect by changing the location of the reading material, so the material is not in that part of his visual field that is impaired.

Defective Word Recognition. Some aphasics use certain words improperly as parts of speech, i.e., *he* instead of *she* or *right* instead of *left* (opposites).

Loss of General Comprehension. To comprehend what you read, you must follow the author's thoughts toward an idea or a conclusion. If aphasics don't understand certain words or have trouble with sentence formation, then it will follow that they will have extreme difficulty following combinations of words, sentences, and paragraphs. Sometimes an aphasic will correctly read all the words in a sentence, but won't be able to comprehend what that sentence means.

IV. IMPAIRMENTS OF WRITING

Poor Hand Coordination. Because most aphasics are hemiplegic, with a paralyzed right side, those who were right-handed have to learn how to use their left hands for writing. They experience many various difficulties, ranging from problems tracing over a circle to copying words or numbers.

Defective Recall of Letter Shapes. Some aphasics can spell but when it comes to writing they can't recall the letter shapes. When they try to write, some letters appear to them like mirror images, or strange symbols. This difficulty applies not only to letters but also may extend to linear or symmetrical forms, and to all copying of objects (i.e., whether copying a house or a person).

Poor Recall of Spelling. Some aphasics have difficulty with spelling orally, or writing. In some cases this is related to poor auditory recognition. They don't hear the right word or sound, internally and externally.

Difficulty with Sentence Formulation. This is the same as the fourth behavior, listed under Speaking, since the same syntactical and rules apply to both.

To further describe the aphasic's language problems, Diagram A shows language pathways on seven different levels, from thinking to speaking.[2] These levels represent progressive thought processes, moving from symbolic to syntactical and comparing the aphasic with the "normal" speaker. These diagrams and statements will enable the reader to put the aphasiac's communication problem in perspective in order to understand the bases of the personal reports which I have studied.

DIAGRAM A
NORMAL LANGUAGE FORMULATION

1. *Internal Level of Awareness* (Consciousness)
Total Impressions, Sensory Images
↓

2. *Internal Level of Thought Schema*
Schematic Formulation of Thoughts:
Conscious of Content, Without Verbalization
Esthetic Components: Judgment, Creativity, Intuition
↓

3. *Internal Level of Language Schema:*
Language Usage
Internal Thought to Sentence Structure
↓

4. *Internal Level of Means of Expression:*
Internal and External Auditory Perception
A. Musical Elements
B. Affective Elements
Intonation, Loudness, Tempo, Pitch, etc.
Interrogative, Imperative, Declarative, Exclamatory Sentences
↓

5. *Internal Level of Word Choice:* (Semantics)
Word Finding, Word Meanings
↓

6. *External Level of Verbalization:*
Pitch, Volume, Tone, Articulation, Word Finding, Word Meaning
Utterance is the response of language in all the above levels.
↓

7. *External Language as a Communicative Social Behavior*
Affects the Person and His Relationships
in His Everyday Life

This starts out with the basic level as: (1) *Internal Level of Awareness,* where consciousness formulates all sensory images or stimuli; (2) *Internal Level of Thought Schema,* symbolic formulation turns to conceptual formulation as schematic and systematic formation of thought occurs (i.e., you are conscious of contents without verbalization). It is at this level where all judgment, creativity, memory and intuition occurs.

On Level 3, *Internal Level of Language Schema,* one begins to place all conceptual thoughts into some syntactical order. When we arrive at Level 3, we must still remember the original thoughts, so we can arrange those thoughts into grammatical sentence structures. In other words, we place our first symbolic sensing into complex syntactical schemes.

On Level 4, *Internal Level of Means of Expression,* we add musical elements such as intonation, pitch, tempo and affective elements, such as sentences or questioning, imperative statements or exclamations.

On Level 5, *Internal Level of Word Choices,* we deal with semantics. We try to find the most accurate word with which to say effectively what we mean. At last, internal thoughts of grammatical and semantical sentence structures give rise to the next level.

Level 6, *External Level of Verbalization.* It is at this point that we utter our first response. This is a social, communicative, behavioral response, made in consequence to the previous five levels of internal formulation. When we make our utterances, we know what we are going to say to the world around us.

The study of aphasia demonstrates that even the most apparently spontaneous speech is carefully formed. The aphasic's main problem with language formulation does not lie in Level 1 or Level 2, but in Level 3, where he first uses language in a syntactical way. The aphasic has lost rules concerning semantical and syntactical use of language. On Level 3, where a person is supposed to create grammatical sentence structures, the aphasic can't; he has forgotten or lost the ability to apply the learned rules of language. The subsequent levels in language formulation involve continuations of this original problem.

Thus, in Level 4, *Internal Level of Means of Expression,* the aphasic now has to add musical and affective elements; not only does he have to think of his initial stimuli and their ordered grammatical, structured thoughts, but he has also to think of the right pitches, tones and volumes that go with that thought.

On Level 5, *Internal Level of Word Choices,* the aphasic has the added problem of finding the right word.

On Level 6, the *External Level of Verbalization,* or responsive utterance, the aphasic has to go through all kinds of mental gymnastics, just to communicate with others. Finally, this brings us to the last stage:

Level 7, *External Language Used as Social Behavior* indicates that the process used by the aphasic trying to communicate is extremely stressful. If the aphasic is aware of his communication disorders, then his behavior is marked by extreme frustration and depression. People often don't comprehend what he is saying, and they ignore or interrupt him.

On this theory there are five levels of language progression before a speaker can externalize a statement. I propose then, that verbalization at Level 6 is not automatic, at all. The mind must work consciously through all of these five levels. An analogy to these problems is to imagine oneself a stranger in a foreign land. You do not know the language, grammar or intonation, or how to order food or how to ask directions. You might pick up some words, but not enough. When you finally voice your first utterance you will make a conscious, error-ridden response, filled with long pauses, incorrect syntactical and semantic usages, poor articulation and wrong intonations.

A native to the language would not comprehend what you were trying to say, so he would be apt to interrupt you or even ignore you. Soon, from all these reactions, you would begin to feel lost, strange and helpless. In time, your behavior might start to change; you might become angry, depressed, frustrated, or even paranoid.

Such is the case with the aphasic. Because of his inability to communicate verbally, he is always in a foreign land. So aphasia is more than a problem of a physical nature. It involves the whole social and emotional being. To the best of my knowledge there has never been an investigation of the psycho-social aspects of aphasia. These are important to understand, in obtaining a global view of communication.

To summarize, the net effect of his behavioral impairments is that the aphasic is especially conscious of and deliberate in his language components. His speech is a matter of special concern, anxiety, and labor. He always has to worry about what he is going to say, how to say it and how to keep command of that which he has already planned. Normal speakers can keep their minds on their ideas to be communicated, and form their statements very rapidly. But the aphasic must deliberately choose his words and then attend to planning how to form, arrange, and speak them. The aphasic's difficulties lead to the conjecture that a complicated act like speech cannot be spontaneous. Speech is more intricate than is generally understood.

All aphasics have impaired language formulation. Several reported that when their strokes first happened, they were without words. They experienced a bombardment of sensations and perceptions in the present only. They also experienced a sense of euphoria and lack of responsibility–like living in a child's world. They felt a lot of things, but did not have words to describe their feelings, either internally or externally.

Finally, a day to a month later, the aphasics studied began to have internal speech. This was frustrating to them, because they now had an internal voice but they didn't have external speech. Most of them reported that the moment they had something to share, something to communicate with others, their frustration hit.

Some of the most frustrating experiences were mental, sequential ones, which involved reported difficulties in recalling rote memory of names, numbers, listings, etc. The personal, or emotional experiences, provoked anxiety minimally, since they were the most direct and concrete—relatively easy to recall.

The moment they gained inner speech, they also developed worries and frustration, because now they could comprehend the past, present, and future. With this, they began to recall their immediate pasts. Gradually, their sense of self-perception began to return, but it had been damaged. The source of their anxiety about communication was their own perception of what they couldn't say in oral expression. That is, their knowledge of memory of language impairments allowed them to project. What if one blocked on a word? What if he should hesitate and not be able to find the right term, etc.? All aphasiacs reported having these protective anxieties. They knew society has norms in speaking, and unless one follows these norms he will be negatively labeled.

What we consciously remember, we associate in words, and record in the memory of inner speech. But words have personal meanings, and must symbolize experiences before they can record memory. This seems to reason that, although they could identify relatives, without inner speech, most aphasics reported having no memory of the past, and they experienced vagueness about the future. Patricia Neal and Helen Wulf indicated indirectly that memory was inner speech. By means of inner speech we sift through life experiences and discriminate among thoughts. But when they began to achieve inner speech, their memories started coming back. And the moment an aphasic was able to understand the meanings of words in thoughts or sentences, again, he was able to analyze or think abstractly.

The accounts I have reviewed show that it is only when the aphasiac can form meaning in at least his inner words that he is reminded of his past and is able to bring together the union of his past, present, and future experiences. Once they began to have inner speech and gave meaning to words, they could go from the concrete to the more abstract. All experiences, past, present and future, began to be linked together in union.

Scott Moss reported his first recovery of inner speech. While taking a bath he began to summarize consciously what he had to say to his doctor. This was the first time since his stroke that he consciously used inner speech. Before this, he still carried out his daily activities. He dressed himself and did other human functions, but without conscious thought.

But the moment he had inner speech, he was able to summarize, remember, and conceive of the future.

Scott Moss also offers an interesting theory about his aphasia. Because he was having such difficulty with his internal speech, he suffered from anxiety. And this, he proposes, interfered with all of his social activities, which diminished because of this. That notion is supported by the facts that he is afraid to communicate in public, to colleagues and friends, but not to his children, spouse, or speech therapist. With the last three he felt confident that they will understand his problem. It is at this point also that the aphasic admits that his speech is not automatic. He knows it is a conscious and deliberate act.

Expressively, speech and writing are conscious and deliberate acts. They are filled with errors such as word blockages, failures of memory, and misspellings. Receptively, the aphasic comes to know he has an impairment in listening or reading or both. He becomes self-conscious of poor retention and poor comprehension. He is unable to discriminate among sounds, and his world seems filled with too much noise. The knowledge of errors produces anxiety, and it is this anxiety that inhibits all his activities.

Helen Wulf, Scott Moss, Patricia Neal, and Eric Hodgins all reported having this anxiety. But at the same time all were determined to overcome it by deliberately taking risks in interpersonal communicative acts. Wulf, Moss and Neal were all very social people before. In order for them to communicate again they had to take risks in different situations. Patricia Neal tried speaking at the Waldorf Astoria. Scott Moss tried teaching again. Helen Wulf tried talking to different friends and some business activity. Even Eric Hodgins, the least social of the three, after months of risky perseverance, led a fulfilling life by becoming a writer again. Determination to risk interpersonal and public communication was a characteristic of all these people. They all believed that because of their determination, perseverance and taking risks, they regained many of their language skills.

All these studies still projected anxieties, which derived from an awareness of the social consequences of their personal impairments. This leads to the observation that society equates speech with intelligence. Awareness of this and protest against it is found in each case history. Society relies too much on its perceptions of individuals and the qualities of their speaking. When someone stutters or speaks with a slur, people generally think that he has diminished intelligence. The aphasic, so conditioned, in turn, begins to believe that he is less intelligent or is crazy.

When they couldn't talk, all the subjects studied reported feeling inadequate, they were crazy, or had otherwise lost their minds. When they had no way of expressing to the world what they thought, they doubted their own intelligence. Yet they had all these intelligent thoughts and explainable feelings in their heads. Both, they and many who observed them, were mistaken; intelligence had not been lost; their means for communicating intelligent thought had become impaired.

This brings me to another conclusion. There is a direct relationship between self-concept and recovery from aphasia. An aphasic's past self-image indirectly affects his recovery. The aphasic will enter more risk situations if he wants to become his former self again. Accordingly, they would be less apt to recover communicative skills because of their memories of failures.

My suggestion is that the self-concept (i.e., what an aphasiac was in the past) will influence recovery. But this is a variable that clinicians, scientists, or laymen have no control over. Aphasia is such a destructive disorder that those who experience it rarely are able to make a comeback to their former abilities, and tell us about its effects.

The way the aphasiac reacts to spoken (or even unspoken) criticisms will influence how he will recover. Also, how the aphasic can take his inability to speak or do anything as he used to, will influence his healing. He will either pine and feel sorry for himself in case of a failure, or he will be determined to make it better, by doing something about it. By risking high anxiety situations and persevering, no matter what, the aphasic achieves enhanced quality of recovery.

Healing is multi-faceted. In addition to the physical and medical aspects, the psychological health of the patient becomes paramount. This also affects the individual's self-concept and validity as a person. His ability to connect with other people is also very important. All the people reviewed reported being very social before, except one. He also was the least aphasic, but he had the most difficult time in recovering. The evidence also implies very strongly that the person suffering from aphasia needs support from another person, whether a sibling or spouse, or just a friend, in order to assure quality recovery. He needs that other person's understanding, and continued presence to help him along. The other is needed to inspire and to motivate him until he is better. The man who had the hardest time recovering was the only person in the group we studied who didn't have it, at first. But in the end he finally did. The moment he had one other person as support he began to make significant improvement in his recovery.

Again, I want to emphasize that aphasia affects the whole personality. All reported this. Aphasia is not like breaking an arm or having an attack of appendicitis; it is something that changes the whole self, the whole being. Accordingly it is a "new person" who must evolve. He must adapt to chaotic new situations with a whole new set of rules. Only when communication is conceived as an interactive, adaptive experience with risks, can the process of recovery from aphasia truly begin.

REFERENCES

1. Keenan, Joseph, *A Procedure Manual in Speech Pathology With Brain Damaged Adults*, Interstate Printers & Pub., Illinois. Copyright 1974. pp. 8-12.

2. Goodglass, H. & Blumstein, S., *Psycholinguistics and Aphasia*, Johns Hopkins University Press, Baltimore, MD, 1973. p 148.

The Plight of the One-Armed Paperhanger

Nicholas Mikula, Jr.

Having had a CVA early in my life was not good for my career. My practice as a plastic surgeon was terminated before I could even begin it. Undergoing certain therapies (which included physical, occupational, psycho-, speech-language, and recreational) have at least enabled me to carry on living as a "normal" human being. Although my CVA was in 1986, I still am recovering my communication and cognitive skills and am still in speech-language therapy. My years of coping with my ongoing emotional, social, physical, and occupational difficulties have helped me grow as a "human being."

"Coping capabilities": an interesting term. One half of my body only partially functions; my brain (whose third ventricle is wider now because of scar tissues in the grey and white areas); and my noticeable limp that will never go away have strained my "coping capabilities" almost to their maximum.

A stroke at any age is difficult to deal with both for the stroke survivor as well as for all those related to him. I had my stroke at the age of 35, in the winter of 1986. I thought I had so carefully dealt myself a good hand by becoming a plastic surgeon. However, fate had marked my deck. In doing so, she had trumped me. As a result of this stroke my professional dreams were swept out from underneath me.

When I had the stroke, the neurosurgeon placed me into a barbiturate

Nicholas Mikula, Jr., MD, was a Board Certified General Surgeon and a Board Eligible Plastic Surgeon when he had a stroke in 1986. As a result of that CVA he is now right hemiplegic with aphasia and apraxia, but is actively involved as a facilitator in a local aphasia community support group. Dr. Mikula is also currently writing and publishing poetry.

[Haworth co-indexing entry note]: "The Plight of the One-Armed Paperhanger." Mikula, Nicholas Jr. Co-published simultaneously in *Loss, Grief & Care* (The Haworth Press, Inc.) Vol. 8, No. 1/2, 1998, pp. 201-204; and: *After Stroke: Enhancing Quality of Life* (ed: Wallace Sife) The Haworth Press, Inc., 1998, pp. 201-204. Single or multiple copies of this article are available for a fee from The Haworth Document Delivery Service [1-800-342-9678, 9:00 a.m. - 5:00 p.m. (EST). E-mail address: getinfo@haworth.com].

coma. When I awakened from this, I knew I wanted three things to function properly. First, my brain; second, my right leg; and third (if possible) my right arm. My diagnosis was a left cerebrovascular accident (CVA) with aphasia due to a thrombo-embolic phenomenon (from a prolapsed mitral valve) which had partially destroyed both sides of my brain. The left cerebral hemisphere (in particular the cerebral tissue supplied by the left middle cerebral artery) was the most affected area.

My wife divorced me one year after the stroke and took our children with her. I was figuratively and literally left out to dry. My parents, who were in another state, housed me, once again. I had to continue my therapies, which included physical, occupational, and speech, while I was living with my parents. While undergoing these three therapies, I had to take my automobile driving test over again to legally allow me to operate a "handicapped vehicle." After completing my physical and occupational therapies I remained in speech therapy.

When my former speech therapist was in the process of terminating my therapy (since she had taken me as far as her abilities had allowed her to do), she suggested that I enroll in courses at an undergraduate college. I registered for a poetry and fictional prose class in the fall semester of 1988, as well as in a non-fictional prose class for the following semester. Boy, was I ever in for a shock. Contrary to what I was led to believe by my former speech therapist, I was not even close to being in a position to benefit from my prose courses. Much to my dismay, I discovered that my cognitive and speech-language skills were not at a high enough level to enable me to function in these courses. The one bright spot in this "adventure" was that my exposure to poetry turned out to be a springboard to my current poetry creations.

That summer, not realizing I was ill-equipped to do so, I entered into a new medical residency–nuclear medicine. Again, I discovered that I mistakenly had prematurely entered into a situation for which I was not prepared. Because my cognitive and speech-language skills were not adequate, I was unable to benefit from this residency program. I was constantly confused. I became angry and frustrated because I did not comprehend why I had difficulty understanding even simple medical terminology and procedures. Through all of my bewilderment, I was fortunate enough to be surrounded by caring and very helpful people. In fact even the chairman of the department (at the hospital where I had been assigned) went out of his way to assist me.

As part of our residency requirements, all of us residents had to write an article to be submitted for publication. I decided to do a case study. Because of my cognitive and language skill limitations, the chairman organized my thoughts into logical units and communicated my ideas into the appropriate syntactical-grammatical structures, necessary for publication in a nuclear medicine journal. A bright spot regarding this experience was that I discovered that I was capable of living on my own, without the presence of family members.

In addition, during this residency, I started to attend psychotherapy sessions because of tremendous feelings of rage and frustrations inside me. My psychotherapist explained to me that the frustrations of everyday life, low self-esteem, and rage can be vented in positive ways. For instance, I could use my computer for venting. And I have continuously done that venting.

As a by-product of my stroke, I found it easier to compose my poetry than to communicate within the logical restraints of prose. Although one can be "abstract" as one can be when writing verse, one indeed needs to have "a foot on the ground" for everyday life. Prose in everyday conversation is a real stickler for precise communication. I sadly realized that I was in no way prepared for even everyday communication.

Fortunately, my neurologist recognized the fact that I could not read even a simple normal sentence. He referred me to my current speech-language pathologist. She has done wonders for me in improving my cognitive as well as my speech and language skills. They are increasingly enabling me to improve my communication and function in everyday living. In addition, she has become my editor for all my poems, letters, speeches, and other writings.

The term "bereavement" has special meaning for me. I wish to describe my emotional reactions after the stroke. It was as though all of my emotional feelings were put into an orbital spin, only to land in an intermingling disarray of feelings. An overlap of hypersensitivity poured into all of them. My sentiments of love and hate managed to get themselves caught up, like a ball of yarn. I used to lose my temper at even the smallest of things. And then I would rage into storms of profanity. In addition, when conversing with people, I could not figure out why no one could understand the meaning of my thoughts.

My current speech-language pathologist is doing a spectacular job. Through a myriad of modality stimulation techniques, she is improving my logical formulation skills as well as my ability not only to communicate better with myself but with other people, as well. In general, because of her therapeutic techniques, my cognitive, memory, and speech-language skills are ever-increasing.

My present more peaceful state of mind has not been achieved without a struggle. As time has gone by, the right hemiplegia still reminds me of where I had been. But I am continuing to make an increasingly more flexible return to everyday life. I can now read simple sentences, do not converse in an aphasic-apraxic monotone voice, and am more easily able to communicate with people around me. Most strangers now think that because my right arm is in a sling, it is the result of a recent accident. My continuing progress gives me the courage to continue to improve for the future.

In general, each stroke is a unique medical problem. Its myriad complications from hemiplegias, aphasias, and apraxias, make each one of its victims strive, if possible, to become a stroke survivor. All of the therapies, including physical, occupational, speech-language-cognitive, and (if need be) recreational should be utilized, if possible, to their fullest.

Perhaps, my poem "The One-Armed Paperhanger" best communicates my emotional adjustment to my stroke.

"The One-Armed Paperhanger"

He had two arms now, only one!
A plastic surgeon
Mind and hands able to create!

Facelifts and nose jobs
Sculpturing the dermis with sutures
Making the skin that much more beautiful

A stroke at an early age
only the Mind working overtime!

His Mind
A sculpture unto itself
Bad from good, hate from love
Fortunately, love will always come out on top!

Now, similes and metaphors
Poems about anger,
Short stories about love,
A "one-armed paperhanger" only in physical
appearance!

The Perils of Travel,
Following a Stroke

Norman Gootman
Phyllis M. Gootman

Although improvements in travel are being instituted more competi-tively than ever, these days, the physically handicapped traveler may sud-denly find himself even more challenged than he imagined. In 1993 I discovered how hard it was to beat the odds, and I learned about the hidden man-made perils of traveling.

In 1989 I had a major stroke (cerebrovascular hemorrhage), and be-came right hemiplegic with very significant expressive aphasia. In fact, I really was not expected to make any functional recovery, following the complications of coma, adult respiratory distress syndrome and metabolic derangements. Nevertheless, I recovered consciousness and have been working towards improvement of motor, speech and cognitive functions, ever since.

A setback occurred in October of 1993 when I had another, albeit smaller, occlusive stroke. Nonetheless, after returning from intensive reha-

Norman Gootman, MD, is Visiting Professor of Physiology and Biophysics, and Professor Emeritus of Pediatric Cardiology at the School of Graduate Studies at SUNY Health Science Center in Brooklyn. He is also Clinical Professor of Pediatrics at Albert Einstein College of Medicine. Phyllis M. Gootman, PhD, has served as Professor of Physiology and Biophysics at the School of Graduate Studies, SUNY Health Science Center in Brooklyn. She also is an appointed Consultant in Pediatrics at Schneider Children's Hospital, a member of the execu-tive board of the American Autonomic Society, as well as on the editorial board of *Journal of Developmental Physiology.*

[Haworth co-indexing entry note]: "The Perils of Travel, Following a Stroke." Gootman, Norman, and Phyllis M. Gootman. Co-published simultaneously in *Loss, Grief & Care* (The Haworth Press, Inc.) Vol. 8, No. 1/2, 1998, pp. 205-213; and: *After Stroke: Enhancing Quality of Life* (ed: Wallace Sife) The Haworth Press, Inc., 1998, pp. 205-213. Single or multiple copies of this article are available for a fee from The Haworth Document Delivery Service [1-800-342-9678, 9:00 a.m. - 5:00 p.m. (EST). E-mail address: getinfo@haworth.com].

bilitation, with the encouragement of my wife, Phyllis, and the passage of the American Disabilities Act, I decided to travel abroad.

You can't allow yourself to be depressed, following a stroke. Since travel always was an uplifting experience, it seemed an especially good idea at the time. I believe that if you feel you will constantly improve, you will. The key is that you have to want to, strongly enough, and keep working at it. My attitude assured my wife, as well, that travel abroad was possible for us.

So far, our travel has been limited to attendance at scientific meetings and conferences at which Phyllis and I are expected to present our research and participate in discussions and committee meetings. However, getting to these meetings and having the necessary equipment available for my special needs at the hotels and conference centers proved to be a major problem. Also, getting around a city, and eating in restaurants became challenges in logistics, as well as lessons in frustration.

Originally, we started by just calling the hotels, chatting with one of the assistant managers, or head of housekeeping in some cases, and being told that all the necessary handicap facilities were available for me. Naturally, we assumed this was the truth. Were we so naive! So, in 1993, four years after the CVA, we planned our first stay at a hotel. We decided to attend the conference of the International Union of Physiological Sciences in Glasgow, Scotland.

We were told that Moat House International was connected to the convention center. We also had been informed the entire meeting was to be held there, and that it was fully wheelchair accessible and equipped for the physically challenged. (Just to make a long story short, *now it is!*) We arrived from the airport in two taxis, one for baggage and one for the two of us, our helper and a colleague traveling with us. The taxi, supposedly equipped to handle wheelchairs, could not manage my chair, which is about two inches wider than a standard wheelchair. The old fashioned Bentley taxis, for which the UK is famous, were of no use to us because they have a very high step into the cab. We needed a standard type car or station wagon, which proved to be not quite so easily available. Then, after all that, the hotel entrance had to be specially unlocked and opened because they were only using a rotating door.

When we finally got upstairs, our room was not adequate. The entrance was too narrow for significant manipulation of the chair into the bathroom, which was not properly equipped. There were some low bars as if for a paraplegic. But even a paraplegic could not have functioned in that bathroom. Rods were in the wrong place, the toilet did not have lift support bars, and no wheelchair could fit under the sink. However, the staff was willing to take direction, so Phyllis became an ad hoc contractor and "subcontracted" to the staff and purchasing office. The bathroom required a tub bench, support bars, change in location of shelves, phone, towel racks, handle in the shower, elevated toilet seat, and bars for support onto and off the toilet. The marble apron around the sink was too low, and required too much effort to remove while we were using the room. However, I was finally able to use the bathroom about nine hours after our arrival at the hotel.

Other problems in Glasgow were not so easily solved. The meeting was not solely at the convention center. Many lectures were held at the University of Glasgow, which was built in 1451, and seemed as if much of it was still from that period. While there were some buildings that were accessible, unfortunately most of the sessions we wanted to attend were not. In addition, local transportation was a significant problem because of the lack of adequately equipped taxis. Even the few special handicap taxis they did have there had ramps and doors too narrow for my wheelchair.

Restaurants were a particularly problem for us, in Glasgow. First, we encountered the predicament of transportation of the wheelchair to the restaurant, and then the problem of getting into the restaurant, itself. Finally, there were steps within the restaurant that made it impossible to eat at certain levels. That meant that the varied types of food we expected to have were not available to us because it was necessary to go up or down steps to reach each specialty level. What was particularly unfortunate was that we were told in advance that the restaurant was accessible but it turned out to be so only at one level, the noisy bar. Because of this unforseen problem, we ended up having most of our meals at the hotel. It was not a hardship from the point of view of food, but it proved somewhat limited as far as menu choices. Because of this we were not able to enjoy much of Glasgow. On the other hand, the Scots are charming people, and they tried to help as best as possible, whenever confronted by our having a problem (e.g., crossing streets).

After Glasgow, we went on to Dublin, Ireland. This city is far better equipped to inform the handicapped as to availability of public facilities, such as museums, parks and theaters. They have a specially published booklet that was extremely helpful in locating restaurants, theaters, etc. But getting on and off the small airplane proved to be another onerous experience. Again, we found that help was available, and the Irish are extremely pleasant and helpful. As before, our hotel had promised us a fully equipped room and bath.

But even here the bath was missing a number of items. At first, there was a question about not doing the necessary construction changes, since it was a holiday time in Ireland. I informed the manager that we were dealing with an emergency, and he must get the necessary people in. He did, and that made the hotel quite comfortable, as far as the room and bath were concerned. However, their restaurant was a disaster! We had to eat lunches and dinner elsewhere. Since the hotel was well outside Dublin, proper, this became a problem with transportation, especially in the rain.

Again the choice of taxis became a major problem. They tended to either be the old fashioned type (with a very high step) or small German cars. Neither could serve my needs. We finally found ourselves describing the exact size of the cars required since the trunk (boot) had to hold the wheelchair, and the front seat leg room had to be long enough. Our hotel was just opposite the University of Dublin, where our conference was scheduled. However, that thoroughfare proved unpassable on foot with a wheelchair. There were a number of roads that fed that artery, and the traffic and curbs made it impossible. Thus, we had to call for a taxi to take us around and across, each time we just wanted to cross the road.

Sightseeing in Glasgow and Dublin was possible because the cities arranged for handicapped accessibility to at least some of the major sights or museums. The leading problem was the logistics of getting a proper taxi to the sites and back. Sometimes we had to send away three taxis before the right size finally arrived.

Now, accessible restaurants or hotels with accessible restaurants can be easily found, using the handicap guide book. Recently, we had good luck at one, which had two different restaurants, both of which were excellent. The handicap bathroom facilities were also fine. I recall that we had the unforseen problem of not being able to use a handicap stall in the men's room because my spouse is a female caregiver.

This can be a significant universal problem, wherever one travels. Even at such a major landmark as the New York State Theater at Lincoln Center we had to go down to the gallery and across to the entrance of Avery Fisher Hall, to find a unisex handicap toilet. You can miss acts with this trip, which also involves a lot of elevator service.

The next meeting we attended was in Seattle, Washington, in the spring of '94. We must have driven the staff at the Society for Pediatric Research crazy with all our calls. We had two accepted presentations at the Society's annual meeting and were eager to attend. Here, we had no problems. Although the prior arrangements took a great many calls, the outcome was superb. The citizens of Seattle should be very proud of their compliance with the Americans with Disabilities Act. Greyhound of Seattle had handicap minivans that lifted me in the wheelchair. While their drivers had to study the notes to set up the brake system, they were cheerful about their shortcomings and managed to get things straightened out. The vans were also large enough to take all the luggage, as well as the passengers.

We stayed at a major hotel in Seattle. Just about everything was ready for us. My wheelchair (electric scooter) was too large for the bathroom, so we were loaned one from hotel security. Since they needed it during the day for visitors, it was brought to us in the evening (or at 6 A.M.) and picked up at their convenience. The toilet support bar was on the wrong side for my handicap, so the next day, another bar was installed for me. The elevators, restaurants, and even the pool area were wide enough for me to get around on my scooter. Taxis were not a problem at the hotel, but could be at a restaurant because we needed a strong man to lift the scooter into a station wagon. The minivan was used for airport service. The sidewalks had cuts so we were able to sightsee way down to the market, and eat at the waterfront. The convention center was a joy. Since there were no unisex handicap toilets, the medical center's bathroom was made available for me. We just had to find a security person to call to get the bathroom opened. Restaurants were accessible including the famous Space Needle. All the hotel restaurants we tried were superb. The staffs went out of their way to help us, and we had a marvelous stay in that city.

In the summer of 1994 we attended a Sudden Infant Death International Conference, held in Stavanger, Norway. This required transfer in Oslo to a small plane. Getting on and off the small airplane presented special problems. But, by now, Phyllis had gotten to the point of faxing our detailed requirements to the travel agents and I was sent back a fax indicating that all was ready for us as far as the hotel, conference center, etc.

Feeling like seasoned travelers, by now, we arrived at the hotel and were surprised to find that things were not as they had stated they would be. While we could manage beds that were too small and not separated, I had to have a bar in the shower for support, as well as bars on the left, next to the toilet. The alleged handicap room we were given also had high door sills between each of the rooms. Initially, they wanted to do nothing to help us, but this was not acceptable. Phyllis convinced the workman that there was adequate space to arrange things in the bathroom of our double room. Apparently the shower wall had no stud supports within the wall to handle a support bar. We found one spot in the corner which had a stud, so we put the bar at that location. He also built wedges to go under the high sills so I could carefully manage to get into the bathroom. I was never very secure about the slope, though. We called the travel agent and got a true shower chair (not a patio chair, which is what the hotel was calling a shower chair). We were also sent a scooter for getting around. And portable lift bars were put in the toilet. According to the somewhat uncooperative woman at the desk, they had not received my fax (sent three months earlier) until the day before. When I asked why they said all was in place, she just shrugged her shoulders.

But the rest of the staff and the people of Stavanger tried to be most helpful. In this city, taxis were definitely not a problem. The taxi service had about nine vehicles that were equipped to lift wheelchairs, or with ramps for the wheelchair to ride up. Although the city is hilly, many of the places we visited were reachable by foot and scooter from the hotel. Unfortunately, because of the hills, most of the restaurants are built on levels with steps, and thus, were not accessible. The hotel restaurant was quite good and, with the staff's help, we did find two others that were accessible. We did have one unfortunate event, though. We were told a sightseeing ship was properly outfitted for the wheelchair, and we could sail out into the fjord. Finally, after five days of run-around, the truth came out. All the ramps were too narrow for the wheelchair, and there was no electric lift. Thus, we were unable to see the major sight of Norway–the fjords. To take the ferry on a return trip up the fjord would have been a 23 hour trip, much too exhausting for both of us. Phyllis was so annoyed that the dentist she had to visit suggested she write to the English page Editor of the local paper. She actually did that, but we never found out what happened to her letter.

Regardless of this annoyance, we must state that the Norwegians were most hospitable. I inadvertently left my cane on a road, during a visit to the local hospital. This led to my having to borrow a tripod cane from them, but we later found my cane waiting for us on a prominent rise in the street. Someone had placed it there, where it wouldn't be missed by the person who had lost it.

Our experiences finding inadequate hotel accessibility, unfortunately, were not isolated ones. In 1994, there was an article in the *Seattle Times* that originally was published in *The Phoenix Gazette*, regarding the upsetting experience of a handicapped man in a New Jersey hotel room. Although it is now more than two years since the Americans with Disabilities Act took effect, according to the article there are still more than 44,000 hotel and motels in this country that do not meet the needs of physically challenged travelers.

On the other hand, in October, 1994, we attended a conference of the American Federation of Clinical Research, which was much closer to home, in New York City. This time Phyllis dealt with the organizers by phone and then rechecked with the hotel. I am pleased to report that both the organizers and the hotel were ready for us. Because of the sex difference between physically challenged and caregiver, we needed unisex single occupancy bathroom facilities. We were concerned about the parking in New York, which is usually a problem.

Well, the major hotel we stayed at in the city had valet parking, and help with the scooter. And a special handicap hospitality room was set aside for our use for the duration of the meeting. The dining room was wheelchair accessible, and the food was excellent. The staff was most willing and helpful. We then attended an afternoon wedding at a hotel in Piscataway, NJ. The manager there also had agreed to arrange for a handicap room to be made available for our use. Interestingly, in both cases the shower-tub would have had to be modified for use by a hemiplegic guest. There was no sliding tub seat or hand bar for support.

AIRPORTS

Back to airports. We have had some very interesting experiences in airports. Let's start with my displeasure with one major international carrier. It was too much trouble for them to seat us together. The physically challenged person had to fly in business class and the spouse in coach. When I wanted help, they ended up having to get Phyllis from her distant seat. We had already traveled across America on other airlines, with no problem to the cabin attendants. We ended up, at increased expense, having to switch our flight to Norway to another airline.

That flight, both going and returning, proved to be most comfortable, with extremely helpful staff. However, plane transfers, both in Glasgow (enroute to Dublin) and in Oslo (en route to Stavanger), led to some hair-raising experiences. The transfer flights were small planes and there were stairs, but no ramps. The staff had ideas of carrying me (hemiplegic, 230 lb., 6 feet tall) up and down these stairs. Each time I thought I would have another stroke right there. This is not the way to transfer handicapped passengers.

Once we were able to use the lift that was used to raise and lower the food carts. Phyllis tried to arrange the same on the return leg of the trip but no one listened. That haul down the airplane stairs was not to be believed. I would imagine those attendants had very bad backs and strained muscles for at least a week or two.

SUGGESTIONS AND HINTS

Basically, we would suggest that, until the travel community is more sensitized to the needs of the physically challenged, one should limit travel to countries where you speak the language. Without the proper precautions, you may be doing construction or at least contracting to get the bare minimum of what you require to function in your hotel room. If you are a large person, stick to bigger cities, with well-equipped airports. Obtain the booklet from the Department of Transportation which tells you your rights as a traveler. You would be surprised at what we are entitled to have available for us.

To have a fighting chance, make of list your requirements for hotels or other needs. Fax it, well in advance, to the manager of the hotel or the arranger of the conference. Do not go to that hotel unless they confirm they have facilities suitable for your specified needs. That way, if you arrive and nothing is set up for you, you have it in writing and can demand that they get it together. Without this, you will not have the necessary documentation to demand your rights and requirements, and can expect trouble.

There are also other resources for information. In particular, the Eastern Paralyzed Veterans Association has a number of excellent booklets regarding rights of the physically challenged. The Consumer Information Center (Pueblo, CO 81009) can supply you with an excellent summary of the various most-used airports, and their facilities. It is called *Acces.5 Travel: Airports, 6th Ed.*, Airports Council International, North America, 1993.

There are a number of organizations that can supply information and help, such as: Mobility International USA in Oregon (503) 343-1284; Society for the Advancement of Travel for the Handicapped, in NYC (212) 447-SATH; and Travelin' Talk Network (800-365-1220).

I learned from experience what to request in advance, when traveling. My personal list of requirements may give you a better overview of what you may find necessary. But remember to fax your list, and have it confirmed in advance by the person in charge, wherever you are planning to travel. Here is my personal list:

Meeting Site

1. Unisex bathroom available at site of meeting (physically challenged individual has opposite-sex attendants, and cannot make use of handicap stall in male bathrooms)
2. Ramp entrance and elevators large enough for oversized wheelchair/ scooter (electric) to reach meeting floors

Hotel

1. Fully accessible entrance
2. Dining room accessible to scooter/wheelchair
3. Hallways large enough for scooter to turn a complete circle

Room

1. Large enough entrance without obstruction blocking the bed (two beds) with table between beds
2. Access to right side of bed with scooter
3. Room with space large enough to turn scooter/wheelchair completely around
4. Closet doors and furniture not in way of electric chair
5. Easily accessible plugs near bed for special mattress pad
6. Bathroom door and bathroom large enough for scooter
7. Room under sink to fit wheelchair or scooter
8. Raised toilet seat with bars for support on left side
9. Tub with hand-held shower spray
10. Bar for left hand, on tub/shower wall
11. If tub then there should be a tub bench so the individual can sit down on outside, swing feet in, and with left hand be able to position in tub for washing. The bench should not block use of left hand for positioning body in tub.

Airport

1. Fully accessible entrance into plane, without steps
2. Unisex handicap bathroom (physically challenged individual has opposite sex attendants, therefore cannot make use of handicap stall in male bathrooms)

SUGGESTED READING

Crowder, Rick, "Planning a trip when the traveler has a disability," *Stroke Connection*, January/February 1993.

Planning a Trip
When the Traveler Has a Disability

Rick Crowder

So you want to plan a trip. No problem. As a matter of fact, planning a trip can be half the fun of taking it.

So you have a disability, too. Again, no problem. You just have a few more things to take into consideration, like accessible accommodations, transportation, and what to do in case you encounter difficulty. That's what my friends and I are here for. Regardless of your disability and regardless of whether you're going across town, across the country, or around the world for business, a wedding, a conference, or a vacation, there are plenty of resources available to help you plan your trip.

Access: International, for example, has a videotape library of accessible attractions around the world if you're looking for some good ideas. And Mobility International USA presents a great book of testimonials and resources. For more good books about disabled travelers' experiences, contact Helen Hecker at The Disability Bookshop. These resources have a lot of accessibility information, too. At the end of this article I'll present the address where you can contact them for more information.

If you already know where you want to go, the next two resources might be very valuable for help in planning your trip. The Moss Travel Information Service will search the files they've accumulated from other travelers with disabilities and will send you all the accessibility informa-

Rick Crowder is Founder of Travelin' Talk Network. He was named the 1991-92 Disabled American of the Year, Clarksville, TN.

Reproduced with permission from the January/February 1993 issue of *Stroke Connection*. Copyright American Heart Association.

tion they have on up to three locations per request. Douglass Annand has written a book called *The Wheelchair Traveler* that lists hotels, restaurants and attractions all across North America found to be accessible by other disabled travelers, too. Or you can just contact me and my friends and we'll be glad to tell you what's accessible in our neck of the woods.

If you'd like to take a group tour to some far away location and leave the planning to someone else, you can contact Accessible Journeys, Evergreen Wings on Wheels or Flying Wheels Travel, to name a few. They specialize in tours for disabled people, and they send tours around the world all the time. Or you can contact me for more companies just like them and even some who specialize in particular locations, activities and types of disabilities.

Just as there are all kinds of different places to travel for all kinds of different reasons, there are all kinds of different ways to get there, too. There are highways and roadways, airlines and airways, boats and cruises, railroads and all kinds of combinations thereof.

For those who want to rent accessible ground transportation or for those who may find themselves needing emergency repairs along the roadways, the "Wheels" section of the *Travelin' Talk* directory presents the most extensive listings available. My friends and I have found many locations for vans with wheelchair lifts for rent, accessible taxi and shuttle devices, van conversion shops, and mobility equipment dealers across North America.

And for those of you who hit the roads in accessible recreational vehicles (RVs) there's a club called the Handicapped Travel Club. For those who ride or drive on only two or three wheels, there's a club out there for you as well. It's called the National Handicap Motorcyclist Association.

When it comes to flying the airlines, things start to get a little sticky. Flying is one of the most difficult means of transportation for some people with disabilities, depending on the nature of the traveler's disability and the availability of ground transportation to and from the airport. You can refer to the "Wheels" section of the *Travelin' Talk* directory for more information.

If you've never flown as a disabled person before, a free booklet by the Eastern Paralyzed Veterans Association will help get you started asking and answering the right questions.

Cruises are a great way to travel. But just as there are differences between cruiselines, there are also differences between ships within the same cruiseline, and differences between cabins on the same ship as well. Contact a travel or tour agency which specializes in travel for disabled people, have taken cruises themselves, and reserves nothing sight unseen. My friends and I have compiled listings of these "special agents," too.

The railroad environment can be the most challenging for disabled people, especially wheelchair users. But, if you rule out transportation via railways you also rule out what might be the most breathtaking scenery you've ever seen, what might be the cheapest and sometimes quickest means of transportation available, and what also might be one of the most relaxing vacations of your life, as well. One book you might find helpful is Robert Reuter's extensive and inexpensive *Wheelchair Users Guide to Light Rail, Heavy Rail, and Commuter Rail Systems in North America.*

So much for accessible accommodations and means of transportation. What if you need a professional travel escort for medical or personal hygiene help on a trip? MedEscort International, Inc. and the Traveling Nurses Network can help. So can some of the specialized group tour operators I've already mentioned.

For those who don't necessarily need a medical professional, but do need a reputable personal care attendant (PCA) away from home, you might want to consider calling an Independent Living Center where you plan to travel. Most of them maintain lists of available PCAs for their local clients and consumers, and they might have just the person you need. My friends and I have compiled listings of Independent Living Centers, too.

If fears about health concerns and possible "what ifs" away from home have kept you confined to a small "comfort zone" or have confined your trips to the United States alone, fear no more. *Traveling Healthy* is a newsletter full of tips and practical health advice about locations all over the world. And the International Association for Medical Assistance to Travelers will help you locate a doctor who speaks English no matter where you might find yourself someday.

In case of an accident or medical emergency, the National Travelers Corporation's PrePaid Air Rescue Service will fly you home via air ambulance from anywhere in the world. (They'll take care of your personal belongings and any family members who might be with you as well.) And to insure access to a family physician who promises to come see you within thirty minutes anywhere in the United States and its territories, there's a Medical Assistance Passport Plan available from a new network appropriately called INN-CARE of America.

But what if you just need to be pointed in the right direction when you're in a strange environment? Say you forgot to pack some important medical supplies, or you get a flat tire on your wheelchair, or your guide dog becomes ill and you need a good veterinarian, or you still haven't found a good, accessible lodging facility or restaurant. No problem. My friends and I are here in case you encounter any difficulty away from home. We're called the Travelin' Talk Network. We're a unique family of people and organizations around the world who have joined hands to make our knowledge of our hometowns available to travelers with disabilities. We've established more than eight hundred contacts in all fifty of the United States, five provinces of Canada, and seventeen foreign Countries around the world. We're still growing by the day, and we're all here to help you in any way we can.

You can find us in the Travelin' Talk directory, the ultimate resource for travelers with disabilities. It's complete with maps showing the locations of our members and has six other sections for the listings of services I've been mentioning. The directory has more than five hundred pages of available resources and was published to help you plan your trips and to lend a helping hand.

For more information send a self-addressed, stamped, business-size (#10) envelope with 52 cents postage for a brochure and a complimentary copy of the Travelin' Talk newsletter.

RESOURCES

Danyaon Coston-Clark
Access: International
P.O. Box 356
Malverne, NY 11565

Helen Hecker
The Disability Bookshop
P.O. Box 129
Vancouver, WA 98666

Douglass Annand
The Wheelchair Traveler
123 Ball Hill Road
Milford, NH 03055

Evergreen Wings on Wheels
4114-198th Street SW, Suite 13
Lynnwood, WA 98036
(800) 435-2288

Davyd Kelton
Handicapped Travel Club
5821 Woodhaven Drive
Corpus Christi, TX 78412

Ten Questions & Answers About Air Travel for the Handicapped
Eastern Paralyzed Veterans of America
75-20 Astoria Boulevard
Jackson Heights, NY 11370-1178
(718) 803-3782

Joan Headley
Gazette International Networking Institute & International Ventilator Users Network (I.V.U.N.)
5100 Oakland Avenue, Suite #206
St. Louis, MO 63110
(314) 534-0475

Robert Reuter
Light Wheelchair Users Guide to Rail, Heavy Rail, and Commuter Rail Systems in North America
Access Systems
P.O. Box 1514
Baltimore, MD 21203-1514
(301) 327-6119

Craig W. Poliner, President
MedEscort International, Inc.
ABE International Airport
P.O. Box 8766
Allentown, PA 18105
(800) 255-7182

Helen Hecker, Executive Director
Traveling Nurses Network
P.O. Box 129
Vancouver, WA 98666
(206) 694-2462

A World of Options
Mobility International USA
P.O. Box 3551
Eugene, OR 97403

Joan Appel
Moss Travel Information Service
1200 West Tabor Road
Philadelphia, PA 19141-3099

Accessible Journeys
35 West Sellers Avenue
Ridley Park, PA 19078
(215) 521-0339

Flying Wheels Travel
P.O. Box 382
Owatonna, MN 55060
(800) 535-6790

Bob Nevola
National Handicap Motorcyclist Association
35-34 84th Street, #F8
Jackson Heights, NY 11372

Karl Neumann, M.D.
Traveling Healthy Newsletter
108-48 70th Road
Forest Hills, NY 11375

National Travelers Corporation
PrePaid Air Rescue Service
5000 Quorum Drive, Suite 620
Dallas, TX 75240
(800) 338-4919

Rick Crowder
Travelin' Talk Network
P.O. Box 3534
Clarksville, TN 37043-3534
(615) 552-6670
(800) 365-1220

International Association for Medical Assistance to Travelers
417 Center Street
Lewiston, NY 14092
(716) 754-4883

Debbie Bratton, C.E.O.
INN-CARE of America
P.O. Box 1204
Clarksville, TN 37041-1204
(800) 933-4627

PART IV
HEALING DIMENSIONS

The Interests and Activities of AARP in Quality of Life Issues and Stroke Patients and Their Families

Helen Boosalis

Nearly 300 years ago John Donne wrote: "No man is an island entire unto himself." The words have become familiar to us–perhaps, at times, even cliché. We often say we're all connected somehow–but perhaps it takes a difficult experience to underscore how important and inevitable our connections with one another are.

This kind of experience visited my family and me when my 43-year-old son-in-law suffered a massive stroke that left him partially paralyzed and

Helen Boosalis, JD (hon), is Chair, Board of Directors of the American Association of Retired Persons (AARP). She formerly served as the Director of the Nebraska Department on Aging, and as President of the U.S. Conference of Mayors. Ms. Boosalis was Mayor of Lincoln, Nebraska for eight years, and has been awarded an honorary Doctor of Law degree by Nebraska Wesleyan University.

Printed with permission from the American Association of Retired Persons.

[Haworth co-indexing entry note]: "The Interests and Activities of AARP in Quality of Life Issues and Stroke Patients and Their Families." Boosalis, Helen. Co-published simultaneously in *Loss, Grief & Care* (The Haworth Press, Inc.) Vol. 8, No. 1/2, 1998, pp. 221-226; and: *After Stroke: Enhancing Quality of Life* (ed: Wallace Sife) The Haworth Press, Inc., 1998, pp. 221-226.

speech impaired. Like my son-in-law, more stroke victims are surviving than ever before. And so the story of my family is being repeated every day by thousands of new stroke survivors and their families.

While stroke remains the third most common cause of death in the United States, 7 out of 10 of the nation's half million annual stroke victims live through the experience. But most of these survivors join the ranks of the more than two million people already disabled by strokes.

Stroke can be a confusing experience for the family. You first notice it when the person disabled by stroke comes home from the hospital. It's then that his or her family discovers that the level of care required is many times greater than they were prepared for.

I saw this happen again and again as patients were released from the rehabilitation center where my son-in-law was being treated. So many of these families were lost and didn't know what to do. Many of them didn't have the kind of resources our son-in-law and his family had to help through the tough months and years ahead: the physical therapy; the speech therapy; the psychiatric counseling for our daughter as well as for our son-in-law; full time help at home to help him out of bed to bathe, dress, and help him with daily exercises and countless other chores. Yes, we were fortunate in that regard, but how many times, I wondered, and still do, what happens to people in similar circumstances who don't have these resources. We were more fortunate, but only by chance.

We were fortunate that my son-in-law's sister is a registered nurse, who heads a trauma unit in Florida. She was able to come to Evanston, Illinois and provide the kind of attention and advice that was so critical in those first weeks of one medical crisis after another when our daughter had to make one life and death decision after another. We have all wondered since why an experienced support system couldn't be organized across this country to give just that kind of support.

We were also fortunate that our son-in-law was young, and that his chances of at least a partial recovery were better because of his age. Their home in Illinois was about a 45 minute drive to the excellent Chicago rehab center where our son-in-law spent almost 5 months following hospitalization. Since he couldn't communicate at all and needed constant care, our daughter had to be with him and away from home and their 7 and 10 year old boys 12 to 15 hours a day, every day!

Again, it was fortunate that at ages 71 and 73 then, my husband and I were able to step in and take over the care of the children and the household to maintain as normal and stable an environment as possible and to relieve our daughter of that added stress. Again, I wondered—how often do people find themselves without that kind of family support, without the kind of friends they had in helping in so many ways—that strong support system that some are fortunate to have but that too many don't have!

Today, with those over 80 making up the fastest growing segment of our population, the number of people needing care will only increase—and rapidly. According to the census bureau, nearly half of all Americans over the age of 85 require assistance with such daily activities as personal care, preparing meals, or doing housework.

We know, moreover, that between 70 and 80 percent of long-term care is provided on an informal basis by family members and friends—and this, too, will increase. More and more of us will be finding ourselves connected in ways we never expected as we begin to care for our spouses, friends, even children. The paradox, however, is that we can also be isolated while connected.

I'll give you an example, a story from AARP's file of stories about the need for long-term care. This is the story of three generations stranded together. It began with a physician, whose first name is Charles. He and his wife Pam, a nurse, invited Pam's grandmother and mother to live with them.

Pam's grandmother had been in a nursing home for 10 months during which she had been hospitalized 11 times. The nursing home costs were rising rapidly. Charles and Pam thought, with three generations in one house, they might be able to give better care and save money.

They were counting on their own medical training to see them through, but then the level of care began to rise and their ability to provide care suffered some serious setbacks. At first they were able to get by with just daytime nursing care for the grandmother while Charles and Pam were at work. Then in 1981, Pam's mother suffered the first of five major strokes that would leave her severely disabled. In 1984, Charles underwent his first surgery for cancer, and Pam's grandmother began to require 24-hour-a-day nursing care.

Pam's grandmother died in 1986 at the age of 95. But then in 1987 conditions worsened suddenly for Pam's mother. She underwent emergency open-heart surgery and, subsequently, suffered a broken leg and had to have one of her eyes removed because of cancer. Finally, Pam's mother could not walk and required around-the-clock assistance.

All along the way, Charles and Pam have encountered the dozens of frustrations that affect the lives of caregivers everywhere. Topping their list of complaints was the fact that their private medical insurance and Medicare proved to be inadequate. When one family faces long-term and multiple medical problems, they often find themselves running short of resources.

Their experience also exhausted them almost completely. After 14 years of caregiving, the isolation and frustration had both Charles and Pam at the point of collapse. They found themselves physically and mentally pushed to the breaking point. Unfortunately, the story of Charles and Pam is matched or exceeded every day by an estimated 25 million Americans– one in ten of us–who are giving care to relatives, friends, or neighbors.

The biggest challenge facing these caregivers is how to balance the load and avoid the paradox of isolation. How does someone care for a spouse or a child and still find time for other responsibilities–their work, their families, their own lives? And I'm not even talking about the simple pleasures of life–like time for oneself or taking a vacation. Unfortunately, the usual and widespread lack of community services and support for caregivers makes this balancing act an overwhelming undertaking and in the end contributes to the isolation of the caregiver.

Let me give you some information to illustrate how much is involved in trying to maintain your balance and avoid isolation.

First, caregiving covers a broad spectrum of services, from bathing and dressing the patient to handling complicated financial matters.

The caregiver's investment of time may range from a few hours each week to continuous, around-the-clock care. In fact, an AAPP survey shows that most caregivers provide some help seven days a week.

About half of the older people in need of care still live in their own homes. And most of these people desperately want to stay where they are. I will return to this point.

Some caregivers face the difficult task of providing long-distance care. A colleague of mine who also serves on the AARP board had to leave his home to be with his 96-year-old mother who lived a thousand miles away. However, most caregivers live within 20 minutes of the person they are caring for.

Only about a third of caregivers and recipients live together–like Charles and Pam.

Although "caregiving" may be a broad and varied concept, the realities of delivering care are by and large predictable. For example, in most cases the caregiver is a family member, typically a middle-aged daughter. For nearly three out of four people with disabilities who are living at home, their sole means of help is a family member or friend. Their caregivers are called on in most cases for physical help because the person in need has physical limitations or is, in fact, house-bound and unable to go out except for medical appointments.

But, perhaps the most striking fact of all–caregivers are seldom trained to handle the one kind of care so many must provide–medical care. Unfortunately, the forecasts for the future only promise more demand for long-term care.

First, Americans are living longer. At the turn of the century, life expectancy was only 47 years. Now it's 75 and climbing.

Second, as I mentioned, the 80-plus age group is the fastest growing segment of the population–and it will continue to be so for the next 30 to 40 years.

Third, our medical technology continues to improve at an astonishing pace. This leaves us with more and more heart attack and stroke victims who survive, but are left severely incapacitated and unable to care for themselves.

At the same time, we will have fewer caregivers to meet this need. The average family size has decreased since 1975. This means that the next generation will bear an even heavier burden in caring for older adults. This poses a double-edged challenge to our country. Do we as a nation want to maintain the best possible quality of life for older adults? And, if we do, are we prepared to commit ourselves to meeting the needs of millions of caregivers?

AARP is facing this challenge on two fronts. We are working to assist current caregivers and planning for the future. Our first effort is to make sure our members, and their friends and neighbors, know about the programs and services available from organizations like the area agencies on aging, local-level support groups like meals-on-wheels, and respite services that offer caregivers well-deserved aid, comfort, and assistance in caring for their aging or disabled relatives and friends.

Our next level of effort is to send AARP volunteers out into the community. These are people prepared to assist people in need. They are responding to Donne's admonition, they are deeply involved with mankind. Our advocates do volunteer work, establish community projects, and hold educational seminars to help older adults and their caregivers make better health-care decisions, including decisions about long-term care.

Nationally, AARP advocates better long-term care in two ways. Our first and most important goal is to reform the nation's entire health-care system. Here we advocate long-term care, along with universal coverage, prescription-drug assistance, and cost containment. These are, for us, the basic requirements of any health-care reform measure that hopes to get our support.

Our second effort on the national scene is called "Connections for Independent Living." This program is aimed at forging partnerships with local organizations that will help make it possible for older persons to remain in their own homes and live independent lives. The concept grew out of our own survey research that showed us an overwhelming majority of our members–fully 87%–wanted to remain in their own homes for as long as possible. Connections for Independent Living is aimed at making that wish a reality for all older Americans.

More to the point, the aim of the program is to find immediate solutions to long-term problems of care, caregiving and protection of the family. It is designed to forge connections between the caregiver and the community and prevent isolation. This goes to the heart of the problem. It is clear to us that the victims of stroke and other disabling diseases and their families need much more assistance than is currently available.

Yes, a stroke–or Alzheimer's or another disease–may remind members of a family how closely connected they truly are. But, now we must find how to connect these isolated–and often struggling–families to the rest of us.

We will work to make connections that will link caregivers in self-help networks. We will strive to make long-term care a part of every plan to reform the nation's health-care system. We will form new community alliances to provide long-term care and respite care services. We will make sure no city or town in America lacks the essential services our older citizens–and younger ones, too–need to see them through their times of need and disability.

In truth, we are not islands. Our needs become the needs of our families. AARP believes in the American family and on interconnection, and the true relationship between all of us. And that, of course, is an obligation on all of us to make sure that no one who is ill and no one who cares for someone who is ill is ever left feeling alone, isolated, "entire unto himself." To the contrary, it is our goal–and has been our work–to make us whole, healthy and entirely together.

That goal can be achieved for my daughter and son-in-law, and for all our families. We all need long-term care protection throughout life. Older Americans and their families need and deserve nothing less.

New Concept in Stroke Rehabilitation

Irving Hirschleifer

During the sixteen years of its existence, the Palm Springs Stroke Activity Center has developed a structured resocialisation program for stroke patients with varying degrees of disability, who still retain the ability to function without full time assistance from a caretaker.

For ease of classification, differentiation, and description, each new client at the Center undergoes a detailed evaluation based on a three stage model of the clinical history of stroke.

The first stage is the acute phase of the illness. The second stage is that of increasing utilization of rehabilitative modalities, e.g., speech, occupational, physical, psychological, and recreation therapies. Over the years we have found it useful to consider those stroke patients who have dropped out of the rehabilitative process to be in the third stage of their illness. These people have ceased their rehabilitative efforts for a multitude of reasons. The patient, or in today's parlance "consumer," or the health professional may be disinterested, having what I like to term exhausted affects, i.e., burnout of emotions. The health professionals may feel that no further rehabilitative efforts would be helpful. Or they may be unaware of a facility such as ours. Further hampering the rehabilitative efforts, the patient may have run out of funds or his insurance company may no longer feel legally obligated to pay the bills. However, perhaps of greatest importance, the patient in this third stage of stroke has no facilities available to further pursue an active, ongoing program for maintenance of his attained

Irving Hirschleifer, MD, has worked in internal medicine, cardiology, clinical pharmacology and geriatrics. He has served as founder, president and member of the Board of Directors of the Palm Springs Stroke Activity Center, and was recipient of the American Geriatric Society's 1975 President's Award.

[Haworth co-indexing entry note]: "New Concept in Stroke Rehabilitation." Hirschleifer, Irving. Co-published simultaneously in Loss, Grief & Care (The Haworth Press, Inc.) Vol. 8, No. 1/2, 1998, pp. 227-231; and: After Stroke: Enhancing Quality of Life (ed: Wallace Sife) The Haworth Press, Inc., 1998, pp. 227-231. Single or multiple copies of this article are available for a fee from The Haworth Document Delivery Service [1-800-342-9678, 9:00 a.m. - 5:00 p.m. (EST). E-mail address: getinfo@haworth.com].

degree of recovery during the second stage, or hopefully, to advance to a higher level beyond his third stage plateau. At the Stroke Center we consider third stage stroke patients as an abandoned and ignored group in need of, and capable of responding to an ongoing organized program.

The Stroke Activity Center was established in Palm Springs, California in 1978 to fill the void in the continuum of rehabilitation of the stroke patient. The Stroke Activity Center has created an optimistic, cheerful and hopeful environment wherein stroke survivors apply and practice what they have been taught by their physical, occupational and speech therapists. This day treatment program is conducted by therapeutic recreation specialists who apply all of the above therapies to individuals and groups in a socially interactive setting.

We employ one health administrator, along with three recreation therapists. There are 70 volunteers who spend varying amounts of time at the Center assisting our small professional staff. We also have among our volunteers several speech therapists, occupational therapists, and a psychologist to evaluate our programs at judicious intervals. There is an internist and physiatrist available for consultations at all times. We have also organized two support groups; one for the majority of stroke patients who are seniors, the second was necessitated by our increasing number of youthful clients and their different generational needs.

At the present time we care for 93 active clients, 46 females and 47 males. The average interval between acute onset of stroke to enrollment in our facility is three to six months; the shortest interval being two months, the longest, ten years.

We strive to achieve one or more of three goals in each client, depending on the underlying morbidity: (1) total or partial removal of a disability, (2) maintenance of an attained level of accomplishment, or (3) slowing the pace of deterioration.

To achieve these goals, individual and group activities are offered to motivate clients to reach higher levels of physical and mental activity. These activities include speech and writing practice, applied occupational therapy, applied physical therapy, and recreation therapy. All of these therapies are directed towards attaining the highest level of independence for the individual concerned. We utilize many standard and accepted techniques plus a number of new methods to attain these aims. While the individual modalities that we offer do not address all of any one client's impairments, we have found that participation in a judicious mix of several programs does result in improvement in speech, perception, cognition, attention span, motor skills and coordination. This results ultimately in a corresponding improvement in the physical, psychological and social health of the patient.[1]

On entering our program, the client and caretaker are evaluated individually, so we may determine which of the various physical, mental and recreational activities are appropriate. These include group exercises, quilting, ceramics, ham radio, dancing, arts and crafts, bingo, writing, reading and speech practice, table games, rap sessions, plus coffee klatches and nutritional lunches. In addition, we have developed several new and quite successful activities.

The first of these is called "Theatre 'N' Me." This is a performing arts program in which clients perform segments of popular musical comedies, which have included *Oklahoma*, *Fiddler on the Roof*, *Annie Get Your Gun*, and more recently our *Stroke Activity Center Follies*. This program has been made possible by the efforts of therapists and volunteers with theatrical backgrounds. Through dance, lip synching, dramatic staging, and memorization of lines, our clients who participate in this program have made excellent advancement in coordination, increasing their sense of self-worth and self-confidence, while improving memory span, decision making, verbal and nonverbal communication, and socialization skills. This program has given a new and wider dimension to the rehabilitation of third stage stroke patients.

A second innovative program is a Radio Theatre in which we utilize available TV and radio scripts, such as *T. J. Hooker* and *The Life of Riley*, to help those who may not have enough motor skills to participate in "Theatre 'N' Me."

Thirdly, we have utilized Pet Therapy,[2] which has been well established for many years. Groups of small animals and their stewards visit the Center regularly. More recently we have associated with the local Pegasus program (an international equestrian group for disabled children), in starting a program for our adult stroke victims. This entails visiting the stables, grooming, petting and in some cases actually riding the horses. They also visit horse shows, and more recently took trips to a nearby race track and a polo exhibition.

Infant Therapy was inspired by a young mother with a recent stroke who had been unable to use our facilities because she could not afford child care for her infant. In order to accommodate her, our administrator set up an enclosed area with clients and volunteers assigned duties for caring for this new visitor. The mother continues to make remarkable progress in her stroke rehabilitation. Unexpectedly, the Center gained even more in return. Our older clients and even some of our most withdrawn stroke patients seemed to gain a new attitude on life, while observing and caring for our new ward. We now maintain a small infant day care center as an addition to our other rehabilitation programs.

We have initiated an "Out & About Program" in which clients are taken to markets and reintroduced to shopping, both individually and in groups. They relearn reading and interpreting labels, handling money, and selecting foods for the Center's lunches. They also help in the preparation and serving of meals at our facility. Other Out & About programs consist of trips to shows, banks, movies, horse races, restaurants and voting.

One particularly enjoyable program developed by our recreation therapists is "Fantasy Cruises" which lasts from six to eight days. Each day one "visits" a different country. Daily entertainment and foods are provided, reflecting a theme for each particular country. Individual and participation have been far beyond our expectations.

"Strokerama," another innovative program, is similar to the disabled Olympics. All stroke clients are entered in some aspect of these games, geared to their disability post-stroke. And everyone wins an award. The pride and increase in self-esteem generated by this program are most remarkable.

The Palm Springs Stroke Activity Center together with our co-sponsor, The American Geriatrics Society, presented in 1993 it's eighth annual one-day symposium for health professionals interested in stroke and its aftermath. This program was designed for all categories of physicians, therapists, nurses, psychologists and administrators. We have been designated a continuing medical education activity for 7.25 credit hours in Category 1 of the Physicians Recognition Award of the Medical Association. The Board of Examiners of Nursing Home Administrators has approved the program for 8 hours of continuing education credit. We are also provider approved by the California Board of Registered Nursing for 8 contact hours.

We usually have 50 to 60 attendees, which at the present time is the capacity of our available space. As many as 40-50% are recidivists, giving testimony to the excellence of our invited speakers and timeliness of the subject matter presented.

Our 1993 symposium was entitled "Comorbidity Problems in Stroke Rehabilitation." Our 1994 program was devoted to the subject of "Stroke Rehabilitation and the Primary Physician." Our symposia are partially financed by pharmaceutical company grants, and those of local extended care facilities. We also obtain partial funding from some of our guest speakers, who are very supportive of our work.

Stroke is a financially and emotionally catastrophic illness. The Stroke Activity Center eases this impact with its no-fee policy. By alleviating the financial stress upon the client and family, recovery is enhanced. This is made possible through community involvement in numerous and varied fund raising events. Examples of these events are an annual dinner dance, benefit and auction, tennis tournament, golf tournament, fashion show and luncheon with raffle, community service groups. There are also individual donations as singular tributes, memorials and recognition of anniversaries, birthdays, etc. Local community support is an all-important factor to both the establishment and continued existence of a center such as ours.

We feel that by using new concepts and techniques that stroke clients find enjoyable, we can successfully improve sensory, motor and cognitive skills, attention span, memory, self management, muscle function, physical fitness and, most important, social integration and quality of life. As the father of rehabilitative medicine, Dr. Howard Rusk said, "It is not enough to add years to one's life, but it is equally important to add life to one's years."[3]

The Stroke Activity Center has operated free of charge to all, since its inception in 1978. Our motto is "Strive and Conquer," and we take pride in the fact that *we begin where others leave off.* We believe there is an increasing need for centers such as ours throughout the country. Although there has been a decline in stroke incidence in recent years, there has also been an increase, due to improved survival, in the number of those meeting the classification of third stage stroke. A specialized facility such as the Palm Springs Stroke Activity Center offers stroke survivors the opportunity of seeking a greatly improved quality of life.

NOTES

1. Bernspang, B., May 1991 "After a Stroke. Restoring Ability of Self-Care." Geriatric Medicine Today, vol. 10, no. 5: 54-59.

2. Fick, K. M., June, 1993 "The Influence of an Animal on Social Interactions of Nursing Home Residents in a Group Setting." American Journal of Occupational Therapy, vol. 47(6), 529-34.

3. Rusk, H. A., *The World to Care For*, Random House, New York, 1972, p. 232.

Conquering Community Barriers: Stroke Rehabilitation

Rosemary Peng
Lori A. Adams
Antoinette Gentile

Being part of community is important to the young or old. Part of our nature is to be social. We want and need to visit family and friends. Many of us even enjoy interacting with strangers. We get out into the community for recreation: to go out to dinner, to see a movie or to visit a museum. Another reason to be part of community is to work, whether for necessity or for pleasure. We also enter the community to fulfill our daily living needs such as shopping for food or clothing, banking, going to the doctor or dentist, laundering our clothes, or participating in religious activities.

The community is a very challenging place to be. It is moving, noisy, changing, and most importantly, unpredictable. This presents difficulty for the rehabilitation process. Lisa Barton and Katherine Black stated in *Advances in Stroke Rehabilitation*, "The environment changes or varies from moment to moment. This factor requires the individual to be constantly reacting to an ever-changing environment. The individual must develop a skill and have the ability to predict or modify this skill for a variety of conditions."[1] The key word they used was "skill." The skill level of

Rosemary Peng, MS, RPT, is Assistant Director of Physical Therapy at Kessler Institute for Rehabilitation, Inc. at Saddle Brook, NJ. She is a member of the American Physical Therapy Association, including its sections on Neurology and Geriatrics. Lori A. Adams, BS, MSP, is Faculty Rehab Director for Novacare, Inc, and was formerly Clinical Supervisor of Speech Pathology at Kessler Institute for Rehabilitation. Antoinette Gentile, OTR, resides in Montville, NJ.

[Haworth co-indexing entry note]: "Conquering Community Barriers: Stroke Rehabilitation." Peng, Rosemary, Lori A. Adams, and Antoinette Gentile. Co-published simultaneously in *Loss, Grief & Care* (The Haworth Press, Inc.) Vol. 8, No. 1/2, 1998, pp. 233-246; and: *After Stroke: Enhancing Quality of Life* (ed: Wallace Sife) The Haworth Press, Inc., 1998, pp. 233-246. Single or multiple copies of this article are available for a fee from The Haworth Document Delivery Service [1-800-342-9678, 9:00 a.m. - 5:00 p.m. (EST). E-mail address: getinfo@haworth.com].

233

functioning in the community requires problem solving and ability to adapt to changing circumstances.

The inability to participate in the community is a common problem for individuals who have a disability. Social isolation that often results can lead to depression or even illness. For this reason, assisting those with disabilities in overcoming barriers to community access is an important and challenging role for rehabilitation. There are many types of barriers for the stroke survivor. Outlined below are different categories of barriers, some which may be more obvious than others.

PHYSICAL BARRIERS

Architectural Barriers. Society is beginning to recognize some of the physical barriers in the community. In fact, due to the recent passage of the Americans with Disabilities Act, many structural changes are being made to accommodate physical limitations in the disabled. It is presumed that curbs, stairs, bumpy sidewalks or grassy areas can be difficult or impossible to manage if a person has to use a wheelchair in the community, or has difficulty walking. Indeed, when one thinks about community barriers, one usually considers those architectural structures which prevent access by wheelchairs. Many in the community think that they can comply with accessibility laws just by installing ramps. In reality, however, physical barriers exist in the community in many unexpected places, and can occur from seasonal and/or weather changes as well as permanent structures.

For someone who has had a stroke, there are many types of physical impairments or problems which can affect safe mobility through the community. Although a stroke survivor may be limited to the use of a wheelchair, often this is not the most common problem. Unsteady gait and balance difficulties may result from paralysis or weakness on one side of the body, or the loss of trunk stability or coordination. Someone with these difficulties may rely on the use of a cane or walker. Mobility is often slower because of the physical limitations or the more complex gait pattern required by the use of an assistive device. The inability to use one arm, sometimes the dominant one, can impair function. The public may not understand how to accommodate for these problems which are less obvious. At the same time, the stroke survivor and their family may not anticipate the barriers which occur because of them.

The community is full of obstacles for the mobility impaired individual. Sidewalks often become cracked by tree roots or other physical forces and can become very uneven. Stairs often have no handrail, only one handrail, or it may end before the top step. Traffic lights can change before a slow walker or a wheelchair user has a chance to complete the crossing. Many drivers are not very patient in the street or parking lot, and do not stop or slow down to let someone cross. Curbs can be excessively high. Doors into buildings are often heavy and close abruptly. A trip to the local supermarket or department store is challenging when narrow aisles are cluttered with merchandise. Individuals with balance or gait impairments need to anticipate raised door saddles and door mats and learn to step safely over them. Even "wheelchair accessible" areas are often inadequate. For example, the "handicapped" bathrooms are usually equipped with handrails, but often do not have elevated toilets or enough turning area for a wheelchair. Elevators are often too small for a wheelchair to fit in, and the buttons can be out of reach to someone sitting in a wheelchair. Entrances to stores and handicapped aisles are often barricaded, preventing someone with an assistive device or a wheelchair from getting through. Rarely is there a bell to call for assistance. Automatic doors for the handicapped often do not work, or the buttons are inaccessible to reach.

Ramps can assist with mobility by allowing people to bypass a curb. However, if they are long or steep, it becomes more challenging. This problem occurs frequently in theaters or sports stadiums. It can be frightening to have to walk or propel a wheelchair down the long ramp. Individuals faced with having to manage such long or steep ramps may not have the courage or endurance to attempt them. Many individuals choose to sit in seats farther back as a result.

Weather. Weather conditions can impede mobility in many ways. When someone has had a stroke, breathing may be impaired because of respiratory muscle weakness. Extreme heat and cold can cause breathing to be labored or blood pressure to rise, even in the person who has normal function. Someone who has had a stroke may be even more at risk for medical complications during these weather conditions. At the very least, harsh weather can affect energy level or speed of mobility. Other ways weather affects mobility include the creation of physical barriers. Even when shoveled after a snowfall, many sidewalks or entrance ways are not cleared wide enough to accommodate a wheelchair, cane or walker. Roads, sidewalks and floor surfaces become slippery after a snowfall or rainfall. The individual who has had a stroke should be taught to anticipate these problems and plan around them.

Crowds. One of the most common hidden physical barriers is caused by fast moving people, especially children, darting out of nowhere, bumping into things and people as they move about. At the very least, maneuvering assistive devices or wheelchairs through crowded areas is difficult. Worse, those who are caught off guard can easily lose their balance and fall.

Other Physical Barriers. Some barriers exist because many persons who have had strokes are limited to performing activities one-handed. It is difficult to physically manage shopping carts, doors or money with only one hand. Reliance on a cane makes it even more challenging because this ties up the hand that is needed for function.

Other barriers exist for those who have poor balance. For example, riding buses, trains or the subway requires a lot of balance. Escalators and elevators require moving at set speeds, good balance to remain upright and coordination to get on and off.

Lastly, those with limited endurance may have difficulty in the community if there are not adequate places to rest. A trip to the bank or post office can test the limits of endurance, especially if there are long lines. Grocery stores do not usually have benches inside, yet it often takes at least 30 minutes to complete the shopping and check out. Even some shopping malls have limited places for resting.

VISUAL AND PERCEPTUAL BARRIERS

Visual and perceptual deficits can have a significant impact on re-entry into the community. However, these problems are not easily understood by the stroke survivor or the family members. The individual often realizes that something is not quite right, however he cannot pinpoint what is wrong. As a result, he masks these deficits, greatly reducing the ability to perform daily routine activities. This can influence functional independence and safety within the community. To effectively conquer barriers which result from these problems, an awareness is necessary of the types of visual and perceptual deficits which can occur.

Vision: Vision is the ability to see. Problems may involve the muscles which control the eye, and/or the nerves from the eye to the back part of the brain. Visual impairments related to stroke can include lack of vision, double or blurred vision, the inability to see half of the normal view when both eyes are open (hemianopsia), or the inability to keep an object focused as it moves nearer or farther from the body (decreased convergence).

Perception: Perception is the ability of the brain to interpret sensory messages from the body or environment into meaningful information. There are many deficits which can occur if perception is altered. These include:

- *Figure Ground:* The inability to distinguish the foreground from the background.
- *Unilateral Neglect:* The inability to integrate and use information from one side of the body (usually the left side) or one side of the environment.
- *Depth Perception:* The inability to judge distances between objects.
- *Spatial Relations:* The inability to distinguish the position of two or more objects in relation to each other, and to oneself.
- *Apraxia:* The inability to plan or execute a task although the concept is understood.

Some examples of how these deficits can impact on function are as follows:

Figure Ground. An individual with this deficit may not be able to find a doorknob on the door or find an item in a grocery store freezer, or on a shelf.

Unilateral Neglect. An individual with this deficit may be hit by a car approaching from the side being neglected. He may become lost due to not seeing street signs, or generally being unaware of only half of the environment. This deficit presents a tremendous safety risk for the individual when navigating through the community.

Depth Perception. Someone with this problem may miss curbs or steps, misjudge footing on an escalator, or misjudge the distance between cars when driving.

Spatial Relations. Someone with this deficit may have difficulty placing a letter in a postal slot or putting money in a vending machine.

Apraxia. This type of deficit can interfere with all aspects of an individual's life. Getting dressed, grooming, eating, opening doors, and folding clothing are only a few of the activities that can be affected.

The biggest area affected when visual and perceptual deficits exist is driving. When driving becomes dangerous, access into the community may be significantly reduced. This inability to drive can lead to social isolation, especially if the individual had been the primary transporter, prior to the stroke.

PSYCHOSOCIAL BARRIERS

Some stroke survivors are confronted with psychosocial issues that may interfere with community re-entry. Some of these areas addressed will not be barriers, themselves. However, the effects of these problems on an individual's functioning can cause barriers within the community.

Self Image. Physical changes are a realistic occurrence following the stroke. This often changes the way stroke survivors view themselves. Some may feel embarrassed by their wheelchair, facial paralysis, or even their brace or cane. Others may feel incapable of performing even simple daily life skills, leading to a sense of inadequacy, worthlessness and dependency. Individuals may respond by isolating themselves within the home, avoiding the community until they are "normal" again.

Fear and Anxiety. Fear and anxiety are emotions that may render an individual powerless against the environment. Some stroke survivors may have a fear of being helpless or dependent on others. They may be overly anxious about their abilities, or fear being unsafe outside the shelter of their home. They may fear the unknown, the "what ifs." There are many opportunities for "failure" in a community setting where an individual is unable to predict or control the situation. Some of these fears are realistic because functioning in the community can be very challenging. However, it is important that these fears do not become debilitating, preventing the person from participating in community activities. Rather, the fears should encourage the stroke survivor to be careful.

Frustration. Individuals may get frustrated over their inability to perform tasks previously done without effort. Anyone who has worked with stroke survivors knows that it is common to hear someone say, "I used to walk so easily" or "I used to talk without having to really think about it." Out of frustration, some individuals just give up.

Behavior. Loss of emotional control, or disinhibition, affects many individuals, post-stroke. They are embarrassed that they cannot control their emotions (i.e., laughing, crying). The lack of inhibition also affects the way the individual expresses him/her self. For example, a person may say something that they would have thought but not expressed prior to the stroke ("Boy she's fat!"). Individuals or their families may not trust these social skills, and limit contacts to home and family.

Insight and Awareness. Some individuals deny that they have any difficulties following their stroke. Often, denial is more pronounced in the "invisible" deficits: perceptual, cognitive, or psychosocial. It is easy to hide or cover up these types of problems. Lack of awareness of these problems leads to an inability to overcome them and improve function. This lack of awareness can place stroke survivors in jeopardy or set them up for failure, upon return to the community. It also prevents these individuals from accepting strategies recommended to increase success.

Society's Bias and Ignorance. Professionals often believe they can predict the hurdles that need to be faced when returning to the community. However, it is difficult, if not impossible, to predict human behavior.

Individuals in the community can be quite insensitive to others' needs and feelings. For example, when crossing a parking lot, despite the presence of walkers, canes or wheelchairs, drivers still choose to proceed without slowing down, and swerve around the individual. At times, questions are directed to the individual's companion rather than to the person, directly. People often refer to the stroke survivor as "they" or "them" in their presence. These actions reduce the disabled individual to an object being talked about, rather than a person being talked to. Comments are made praising the companion for "taking them out." A barrier occurs when the stroke survivor stays home to avoid these comments and public reactions.

COGNITIVE BARRIERS

Cognitive difficulties may give rise to barriers for stroke survivors, once they are back in the community. Often, these barriers, like the psychosocial ones, may be easily overlooked by the stroke survivors and significant others.

Attention/Concentration. Some people demonstrate difficulty attending to or concentrating on an activity, following a stroke. Some are distractable, which means that even when able to attend, their attention very easily can be interrupted by noise, signs and other visual or auditory stimuli in the environment. If a person becomes distracted while crossing the street, for instance, he may stop and stare, which puts him at risk for getting hit by a car. In a grocery store, a distracted person may steer his shopping cart into a display, or another person. Cluttered stores and crowded areas are difficult barriers for people with attention or distraction problems.

Sequencing. Someone who is unable to sequence steps to perform an activity will face a challenging barrier. The person may find herself at a halt in an activity and may not be able to determine what to do next to complete the task. For example, a person may go to the post office to mail a package. The clerk tells her she has to fill out a form and shows her where the form is located. The person goes to the counter to fill out the form and completes it. However, she does not know what to do next because she has difficulty sequencing steps to complete an activity, and no one has provided her with direction beyond this step.

Problem-Solving. Some people exhibit difficulty with problem-solving, following a stroke. If the person previously discussed had good problem-solving skills, she would ask someone for help. However, if she lacks these skills, she may just stand there or may leave without completing the task. There are many situations that arise daily in which people have to problem-solve or make decisions. Such situations include driving to a store and finding it closed, running out of money when shopping, or figuring out how to carry something when walking with a walker.

An example of how difficult it can be for someone who has difficulty with sequencing and problem-solving occurred when a group of patients went to do laundry at a laundromat. One post-stroke patient walked around for 25 minutes, unable to figure out which step to do first. He was not able to begin washing his clothes until the therapist stepped in and cued him. If someone has a problem with these cognitive abilities, even mailing a letter or grocery shopping could be a tremendous task.

Memory. This can also be affected, following a stroke. Short-term memory impairment can become an obstacle for any person who performs activities in the community. In fact, this type of memory deficit can affect every facet of a person's life. For instance, a simple situation such as going to the doctor becomes very challenging. First, the person has to recall the date of the doctor's appointment. Maybe he used a calendar to mark down the date of the appointment, checked daily and knows that today is the appointment. He calls for a taxi. The taxi driver asks for the address and he responds that he can't remember. Without consistently using memory strategies, such as association, or compensatory techniques such as journals, notes and calendars, someone with short-term memory problems would have difficulty with what most people ordinarily consider an easy task.

Pragmatics. Another barrier a person may be confronted with in the community is called pragmatics. Pragmatics is described as social behavior and communication. Sometimes after a stroke, people demonstrate inappropriate judgement in a social situation. "One should not assume that patients are always in control of their behavior because, in the case of severe cognitive impairment, they are not."[3] For instance, consider the person who strikes up a conversation with a stranger at a store, and holds up the line of shoppers. He does not realize that the listener is not interested and is trying to get away. Another person with pragmatic difficulties may demonstrate rude behavior towards others. Sometimes these people are confronted with barriers that may create safety issues for themselves or their families. What if they offend the wrong person? The possible repercussions are endless, as one can imagine. The least that can occur is embarrassment.

COMMUNICATION BARRIERS

Another barrier, which is less obvious, is due to impaired communication skills. Whether the stroke survivor has aphasia, dysarthria or a cognitive problem is not important, here. What is of consequence is that the general public often lacks understanding of communication difficulties. Therefore, the person with this kind of impairment may not be understood, may not get assistance when requested and may even be ignored. Impatience is possibly the strongest barrier someone with a communication impairment must deal with in the community. After all, we live in a very impatient society. Clerks, receptionists, food service employees and other customers are all in a rush. Who has the time to wait for a person with aphasia to get a word out, or a person with dysarthria to speak clearly, let alone wait for someone to recall the name of the product he is searching for? People often become impatient or uncomfortable with someone who has difficulty communicating. One patient had the phone hung up on him when he tried to order pizza. Another had a store clerk walk away from her when she tried to ask a question. People who use some alternate methods of communication, such as augmentative communication devices, gestures or communication boards are often confronted with the same barriers.

REHAB PROGRAMS TO ASSIST
IN DEALING WITH THESE BARRIERS

There are a variety of rehab programs and ideas that are available to assist stroke survivors and their families in dealing with these barriers. The individual who has had a stroke and his or her significant others should become aware of these barriers, so they can anticipate obstacles and be prepared to manage them.

In general, therapists attempt to simulate real-life situations in the clinic. Occupational therapists have had a history of training in activities of daily living (ADL) and work skills. Recently, physical therapy has incorporated the use of more functional activities into the traditional types of therapies. Speech pathologists have also been encouraged to treat in more natural settings than a quiet, isolated office. However, training in real life skills will always be incomplete unless the therapists or health care providers understand the requirements of community life and the barriers which are so prevalent in society. For example, patients are often trained to use the handrail on their unaffected side, when ascending or descending stairs. In the community, however, there are many places where there is only one railing, or even none. Patients who anticipate returning to the community should practice stairs with all combinations of railings, so they can go out wherever they like. This is just one example of the many scenarios the rehabilitation team must consider for the patient.

One program available at some rehabilitation clinics is a day/weekend pass program (or functional trial visit). The rehabilitation team may recommend a patient for a pass over the weekend, either for the day or overnight (if insurance coverage allows). This should only occur after the family has received adequate training. The day pass allows the family to practice with the patient in their home environment, prior to the actual discharge from the hospital. Often, the family may notice difficulties with a thick carpet, a raised door threshold, or in understanding a person's request to use the bathroom. These trial visits are helpful, not only in assisting the rehab team in identifying areas that need attention prior to discharge, but also in preparing the family for discharge. The visits will be most beneficial if the patient or the family provides feedback to the treating team so that therapy can be geared towards specific problems.

A new approach to rehabilitation is to try to bring the community to the rehabilitation clients. Some facilities throughout the country have set up areas where community-like stations are housed within the rehabilitation or hospital facility. These simulated environments are often referred to as "Easy Street" or "Independence Square." These environments have the advantage of providing community-like barriers and challenges within the protective environment of the clinic. They are designed to give the patients the opportunity to practice different physical, perceptual, cognitive and communication tasks, while the therapists are present. The area can be designed to match the types of activities the patients would experience once they went home. Some examples of the types of simulated environments available are a bus, a grocery store, a restaurant, a car, a public telephone, different types of door entrances, an apartment, different ground surfaces (rock, brick, carpet), steps of different heights, and a cross-walk with an electric signal. Therapists who have access to these areas are encouraged to simulate realistic community challenges.

Although these fabricated environments are challenging, it is still important to take patients into the actual physical community. Here there are challenges that cannot be reproduced in the clinic, such as moving vehicles or people, noise, unexpected construction, etc.

Patients are required to cross busy intersections, manage the physical terrain, complete purchases, make decisions and communicate/converse. Another program that some rehabilitation centers have established is a community outing program. Patients are taken out into the community by bus or van, and expected to perform activities as independently as possible. At some clinics, these are interdisciplinary approaches to the functional training of patients. Speech-language pathologists, occupational therapists and physical therapists often make up the teams. Patients are encouraged to problem-solve on their own so that they identify their own solutions to barriers in the community.

For the younger stroke patient, vocational and educational support is necessary for community re-entry. Vocational rehabilitation or industrial medicine departments can assist in preparation for returning to work or school.

Outpatients have other opportunities for training. A big advantage is that they are already functioning in the community and can discuss with the therapists the actual problems they are encountering. While inpatients can only guess at the needs they will have after discharge, the outpatients know what their needs are, first hand. Therapists can concentrate on those skills needed to manage in the community. Some outpatient departments also have the capability to organize community visits in their facilities. They may also achieve this through community outing programs. Outpatient therapists also have gone with their patients to work settings to perform job-site analyses, which give them information about the physical and cognitive requirements of the job. This type of evaluation can also include the use of public transportation.

If a stroke survivor is receiving home therapy, community activities should be part of therapy, as often as possible. Therapists, patients and their families or caregivers can perform therapy outside the office. For example, with the physical therapist the client can practice the physical components, such as door entrances, stairs, sidewalks, curbs. With the occupational therapist and speech pathologist, he can practice problem-solving, communication (i.e., with neighbors), or managing in distracting environments.

Another important program to assist the stroke survivor in reentering the community is an automobile driving program. Before resuming driving after a stroke, an individual may be required to be retested. Many rehabilitation centers have driving programs within the occupational or physical therapy departments. Not only will they test for safety, they also identify the need for special controls to accommodate any weaknesses. Since the laws vary from state to state, it is important to find out the requirements for returning to driving.

SOME SOLUTIONS FOR OVERCOMING VARIOUS BARRIERS

Physical Barriers

1. Be aware of weather conditions (heat, cold, ice, rain, humidity, etc.) and how it affects safety. Know how it can affect the person's physical and medical condition.

2. Before going out, consider the abilities of the companion as well. Make appropriate choices:
   a. Ask for assistance.
   b. Plan rests as you are going up or down a ramp or stairs (i.e., put on the wheelchair brake to rest a few minutes).
   c. Use the wheelchair for distances if necessary. Some malls and amusement parks have them to rent if you don't have your own.
3. Go early, before crowds build up, if this is a problem.
4. Leave early, or wait until the crowd leaves (i.e., at a movie).

Psychosocial Barriers

1, Family and friends should accompany and encourage for support, provide positive feedback.
2. Start out with simple, enjoyable trips (i.e., movie or family visit before grocery store).
3. Make use of supportive counseling or support groups.
4. Acknowledge fears and frustrations. They are real and a normal part of recovery.
5) Family, friends and health care providers should be careful not to make punitive statements (i.e., "It's ridiculous that you feel that way").
6. Allow the person with the stroke to answer questions from servers or strangers, even if the companion is the one being addressed.
7. For the person who denies problems: safety is the main issue.
   a. Assist without confronting. Don't say "You need my help." Instead, suggest an alternate way to perform the activity.
   b. Therapists sometimes need to let them fail within safety limits to facilitate awareness.
8. For the caregivers: check out the availability of respite care, or make use of other family members or friends to provide periodic breaks.

Cognitive Barriers

1. For someone who is distractable, avoid crowds or busy times.
2. If crowds are unavoidable, accompany someone who is distractable, to ensure safety.
3. For someone who has sequencing problems, write down steps, or talk this through, prior to doing the activity.
4. For someone who has memory problems, use memory techniques. (We all use memory techniques!)

a. Write it down (task, list, phone number, address, etc.).

b. Have paper and pen handy and in various locations (pocket, purse).

c. Don't say, "Don't you remember . . . ?" but rather encourage when they do remember.

5. When someone has pragmatic difficulties, the companion should not be embarrassed. Remember the problem is due to the injury.

a. Lability: use strategies taught by a therapist (i.e., three deep cleansing breaths–in nose, out mouth).

b. Inappropriate comments: redirect away from the situation.

Communication Barriers

1. Persist with the communication, encouraging use of any strategies to increase efficiency.
2. Educate the community by exposure to communication difficulties.
3. Become a regular! The more often you go, the quicker they become familiar and increase their understanding.

STRATEGIES FOR CLINICIANS

Health care professionals can help make the transition from hospital to home/community less threatening by incorporating the following tips into their programs:

1. Practice, practice, practice–different surfaces, carrying items of various sizes and weights, opening doors with diverse handles, weights, widths, etc.
2. Listen to your clients. Find out about their lifestyles and the things that are important to them. Many times, we get caught up in our own goals and may miss addressing the client's goals.
3. Validate feelings. Let them know it is okay to be frustrated, angry, upset. It is part of the "healing process."
4. Encourage clients/families to be active participants in the rehabilitation process (attend treatment sessions, ask questions, etc.).
5. Make the practice environment as realistic as possible–progress from quiet to noisy, empty to crowded, still to moving and busy.
6. Reinforce with clients and families that they are never alone; professionals are available as resources, even after therapy ends.
7. Encourage clients/families to get out into the community.

8. Be educators to the public, to minimize ignorance and bias.
9. Encourage clients and families not to give up. Reinforce that life following a stroke can be very productive. They may need to perform activities in a different manner, but most times they can be completed successfully by using assistive/adaptive devices.

Lastly, it can't be stressed enough that as a family member, significant other, caregiver or professional, you need to allow the stroke survivor additional time to complete an activity. No matter how frustrating it is to watch, try not to constantly rescue. Be supportive and encouraging.

In summary, there are many kinds of barriers in the community for the stroke survivor to contend with. One of the reasons for their continuation is that the public has not been educated about their effects on the disabled members of the community. Our hope is, as more individuals with disabilities re-enter the community, society's bias, ignorance and insensitivities will disappear, offering a welcoming place for all individuals.

Think about all these many kinds of barriers. Only by challenging and making them more noticeable will society ever break them down.

NOTES

1. Barton, L.A., Black, K.S.: "Learning Treatment Strategies Applied to Stroke Rehabilitation," in Gordon, W.A. (ed): *Advances in Stoke Rehabilitation.* Boston: Andover Medical Publishers, 1993.

2. Siev, E., Freishtat, B., Zoltan, B.: "Perceptual and Cognitive Dysfunction in the Adult Stroke Patient" Chapters III-V, VII, and Appendix E. 1986.

3. Tellis-Nayak, N: "The Challenge of the Nursing Role in the Rehabilitation of the Elderly Stroke Patient." *Nurs Clin North Am* 21: 339-343, 1986.

Surviving a Stroke:
The Miracles of Science and Spirit

John Holbrook

This essay has a slightly different emphasis. Although there is tremendous value in the approach of modern rehabilitative medicine, I would like to present an unconventional point of view. I am a physician in emergency medicine, with 14 years of experience. As an internist, I was always depressed having to deal with strokes. I think that was because we physicians can tend to model ourselves on God. Despite this bravura, we have had very little impact on stroke, at least prior to the last 15 years.

People suffering from a stroke don't heal dramatically fast. Historically, hospitals have admitted patients with strokes, and three weeks later without much progress, sent them home. We really didn't get that infallible feeling that physicians like. But now we have a tool that can make a profound difference. Most of the time a stroke manifests itself by an absolute loss of control. In a sense, this story is a research project, also without any controls, and with an experimental group of just one. I guess one could say that this is not exact science.

I am a medical doctor, and will illustrate an important contrast between a scientific and a spiritual approach to stroke. My story starts on February 28, 1993 when I was in Albuquerque, on the way to present a paper at a national science convention on artificial intelligence. While still at the airport I received an emergency phone call. I discovered that my wife, in

John Holbrook, MD, is Director of Emergency Medicine at Mercy Hospital in Springfield, MA. He was a student of philosophy and theology before taking his MD at Harvard, and is a member of the faculty at University of Massachusetts Medical School.

[Haworth co-indexing entry note]: "Surviving a Stroke: The Miracles of Science and Spirit." Holbrook, John. Co-published simultaneously in *Loss, Grief & Care* (The Haworth Press, Inc.) Vol. 8, No. 1/2, 1998, pp. 247-251; and: *After Stroke: Enhancing Quality of Life* (ed: Wallace Sife) The Haworth Press, Inc., 1998, pp. 247-251. Single or multiple copies of this article are available for a fee from The Haworth Document Delivery Service [1-800-342-9678, 9:00 a.m. - 5:00 p.m. (EST). E-mail address: getinfo@haworth.com].

her forties, had just had a subarachnoid hemorrhage, and I had to turn around and fly right back. While on the return flight I kept telephone contact and was kept informed of a worsening situation, complicated by respiratory arrest and four hemorrhages. In the stroke world, it doesn't get much worse than that. I was at 40,000 feet, with problems too distant and difficult to solve immediately. It was just impossible to make any decision that could make a difference. I felt alone and terrified.

When we encounter stroke we can deal with it by responding with sadness, grief and loss of control. But we also have statistical models in which relationships must be proven. This has contributed an immense advantage to the study and treatment of stroke. Although I was a scientist, the procedure I had been trained to observe was of no help at all, at the time.

Now, I want to contrast that scientific approach with a spiritual one. Two separate readings from religious traditions describe the human reaction to a terrifying experience. In the Jewish tradition, on Hoerap, the Mount of God, Elijah came to a cave and spent the night there. Then the Lord came to him asking why he was there. "The Israelites have forsaken your covenant, thrown down your altars, killed your profits by the sword, and I alone am left. And they are seeking my life to take it away." The Lord said, "Go out and stand on the mountain, because I am about to pass by." There was a great wind so strong that it split mountains and rocks, but the Lord was not in the wind. And after the wind there was an earthquake, but the Lord was not in the earthquake. And after the earthquake a fire, but the Lord was not in the fire. And after the fire an emptiness of sheer silence. When Elijah realized this, he became terrified, and wrapped his face in a mantel.

The second reading is parallel, from the Gospel of Mark. "Jesus took with him Peter, James and John and led them up a high mountain. And Jesus was transfigured before them and his clothes became dazzling white, such as no one on earth could bleach them. And Elijah appeared with Moses." At that point Peter could not even speak, because he was so terrified.

These passages illustrate our all-too-human reactions to terror. The encounter with my wife's stroke while I was in a plane at 40,000 feet, was such an experience. I was totally helpless and frustrated, and tasted the fear of confronting a loved one, who is dying. I don't know of any scientific approach to such an experience.

The sudden overwhelming reality of stroke immediately cancels all our plans and strips away all our myths. Things went from bad to worse with my wife's condition. She remained in a coma for four and one-half months. During this time I became aware that I had lost about 20 pounds, and wasn't sleeping well. As a physician, I realized that this was not good, so I called my friend, Bill Kutscher, and said I was not quite sure what to do. He quipped that I would gain it back, and the process would be much more pleasurable than this, so better things are ahead. About my disturbance, he added that we should take this as an opportunity to write a book, together, about stroke. "At least, if it has to go on, let's make some fruitful use out of your sleep deprivation."

There was an immense benefit for me, being able to talk to somebody who has been through it before, as he had. This allowed him an objectivity and even humor that I could not possibly have, at that time. As we spoke about advancements in the science of medicine, I sensed that they were not sufficient, in themselves. I began to realize that there could be no substitute for the role of the healer. In many traditional cultures, that person is someone who has already experienced the pain, and understands how to help.

I saw another demonstration of this in the actions of the neuropsychologist at my wife's rehabilitation center. He spent many hours going through her specific problems. In a sense, her brain was a very complex computer network, a parallel processor with a malfunction. We both felt frustrated by our inability to find the right answers. At that time, my wife was still unable to walk, and we all were very upset by this. But then he said, "Don't worry too much about that. I was raised by paraplegic parents." That statement had a profound effect on me.

The fact that this person had been through it before seemed as important to me as any theological or scientific point. I had been deeply affected, trying to understand and accept the reality of stroke. In a previous stroke she had been paralyzed by neuromuscular blocking agents which didn't wear off when they were withdrawn. We didn't know if she could hear then, and was listening, or if she was paralyzed.

I made a decision that at this point she shouldn't be alone. We arranged to have somebody sit with her around the clock, for 18 weeks. Ultimately that involved 45 or 50 people, all volunteers. It is amazing what happened in that process. People read to her, sang to her, prayed with her, played the violin, did her nails, applied her make-up, cut her hair, and talked to her, as if she was listening and completely understanding them.

I am not a real believer, but I called some treatments like crystal therapy "mumbo jumbo magic." I have always been somewhat skeptical, and didn't have too much hope in this, either. But when she finally woke up she thanked them all! She really remembered all the things they had said to her, during that period. Despite my former pessimistic attitude, this proved to me the immense value of caregivers and their healing potentials. There is a very great effect on stroke patients, of having family and friends keep them active company, not just sit with them. This should be an excellent example to ICU nurses.

This illustrates a major difference between mystical and magical thinking. In magical thinking we believe that somehow, being there talking to a person in coma, we are going to make a difference. Our words are going to help make them better, and our prayers are going to have good outcomes. In mystical thinking, however, all we do is sit on that mountain with Elijah, and open ourselves to the mystery, covering our face with our mantle because we are so terrified.

I am vice president of the hospital where my wife was, and the staff worked hard to take care of her. But since this is a Catholic hospital we had many chaplains floating about, offering pastoral care. Since she had a subarachnoid even a cough could be a fatal experience, so I set a big sign outside, "No Chaplain." But, our pastor came in, anyway, and the ICU nurses said, "Throw him out." He responded by declaring, "You are not throwing me out, I am Father Jim Clark." And he walked right in. At this time, my wife had an intercranial pressure monitor that was charting her dangerously high pressure.

Entering the room, Jim said, "Greta, I am here. And, the ICP dropped right down. He sat with her for about 30 minutes, then he got up and said, "I've got to go, Greta." And the ICP started to go back up, again. Then he added, "But don't worry, I will be back again and you will be with me in my prayers." And her pressure then went back down!

When he started out of the door, the ICU nurse said, "I don't know who you are, mister, but you can come back here any time." I am not making an advocacy for some theological argument about the power of prayer. What I am saying is that there is a reality here that transcends the categories and attempted explanations of control groups and statistics. We really don't understand why this happened to her, but it did make a big difference.

One of the most difficult things dealing with the stroke was explaining to my kids, ages nine and eleven, what happened to mom. I think I really was explaining it to myself. My eight-year-old son was in a play at school about St. Nicholas, of northern Prussia, who saved young children from terrible, terrifying things. My wife had worked on the play and now we hoped that she would heal enough in time to be able to see the performance. So everyone decided we would transport her to the school and present a special edition of the play for her.

But she wasn't well enough to do this. Twelve weeks went by so we decided to bring the play down to her, at the hospital. A clip from our local television news said: "A boy brought joy to his hospitalized mother today as he and his second grade class performed a school play right in the hospital. Eight year old James Holbrook and his classmates at the Hartbrook School in Hadley acted out the play at the Mercy Hospital Weldon Center. Nearly four months ago, James' mother, Greta, had a brain hemorrhage. Today, doctors say that, miraculously, she was able to watch her son perform. The teacher had written the play and chose a very special part just for James, who really needed something for his courage. He was given a line that says, 'Take heart good brothers.' Just being able to speak these words in public somehow gave him the strength and courage to go through this very difficult time."

Now, my wife can speak again, and says that the teachers and parents at the school had been just wonderful. Uplifted by her young son's performance, she improved daily and started to walk on her own, not long after that. What I am describing is a spiritual event that really doesn't have a scientific explanation. But it is a reality, nevertheless.

With her kind of hemorrhage the incidence of mortality is four out of five. The chance of walking again is about one in 1,000. The odds of reaching her level of function are about one in 10,000. Now, I would say that there is some miracle here, an exciting encounter with the tremendous mystery of healing.

Last month my wife took a vacation alone to St. Lucia. Now she is driving again, and is reading a book by Stephen Hawking on the philosophy of time. She is doing well. This is a message of hope that after a stroke, nothing truly of value need be lost. Miracles do happen, well apart from all our medical and scientific documentation and experience.

Self-Empowerment in Healing

Wallace Sife

The recovery one makes from a stroke is very different from the kinds of healing most people are familiar with. Since certain brain cells have been permanently disabled, rehabilitation depends on any new adaptations the brain can make to compensate for this destruction. When it comes to physical rehabilitation, some patients are more fortunate than others. But healing now involves more than just the physical self. A stroke traumatically alters the whole person, for the rest of his life. There can be no going back.

We must be concerned with more than just the maximal return of motor coordination and functions. The impact of a stroke is far too profound for us to accept simplistic or dogmatic solutions. We are only now just beginning to realize the extent of the damage that can be caused. The brain is powerful beyond our measurements; it is also the center of sentience. Every aspect of behavior and personality is physically defined here. Some say that the soul itself resides, somehow, within the myriad configurations of this fantastic organ.

The whole person must adapt to the intimate insult of a stroke, and for this an individual holistic recovery program is the best course possible. Grim reality demands an awareness of all the factors involved in what we generally refer to as healing. To focus on only the physical component is as inadequate as it is misleading.

Wallace Sife, MA, PhD, MS, is a published poet, humanist and a psychologist in private clinical practice in Brooklyn, NY. He has specialized in learning disorders, holistic behavior modification, poetry therapy and biofeedback. Dr. Sife is currently at the forefront in developing the field of pet bereavement, and writes in a wide number of other areas.

[Haworth co-indexing entry note]: "Self-Empowerment in Healing." Sife, Wallace. Co-published simultaneously in *Loss, Grief & Care* (The Haworth Press, Inc.) Vol. 8, No. 1/2, 1998, pp. 253-264; and: *After Stroke: Enhancing Quality of Life* (ed: Wallace Sife) The Haworth Press, Inc., 1998, pp. 253-264. Single or multiple copies of this article are available for a fee from The Haworth Document Delivery Service [1-800-342-9678, 9:00 a.m. - 5:00 p.m. (EST). E-mail address: getinfo@haworth.com].

Healing is a multifaceted process. It is holistic, and intimately involved with every aspect of the patient's life. Traditional Western medicine is only just beginning to grasp the relevance of this complexity. Aside from the great physical help that doctors and other health professionals can offer, this fuller dimension of healing ultimately is powered from within the mind.

In growing into adulthood, our awareness becomes so involved with the busy-ness of approval and everyday strategies that we lose sight of the simple blessing of being alive. In a thinking-oriented world, as opposed to a feeling-oriented one, we are trained to look at the concrete and physical values of things. Caught up in the rush of modern existence, we forget how to be centered, or internally aware. When contact is broken with our innermost selves we lose an important perspective on the limits and values of our existence. It is generally accepted that if something cannot be perceived or measured physically, it doesn't exist. We sacrifice a precious part of our humanity in this headlong rush into the frenzied world outside ourselves. But it is never too late for a personal transformation.

Following the crushing private trauma and tragedy of a stroke, a great change takes place. It becomes necessary to determinedly fight one's own way out of this overwhelming flood-current, and gain a psychological awareness of one's new life situation. Since humans are imperfect, our own fears and inexperience can become an incumbrance. Before we can ever really heal, it is necessary to spiritually modify this distortion of personal perspective. My use of the term "spiritual" here implies no mystical connotations. It refers to the sense of personal psychic awareness and wonder that is latent, in different degrees, in each of us.

At first, and in so many ways, the stroke patient's mind is barricaded from the rest of the world. He is locked into his own head, often unable to express his thoughts or feelings to anyone else. Despite our best intentions, the intensity of the resulting emotional trauma can never really be understood by anyone who has not undergone this terrifying experience. The various ravages of stroke are always devastating to the self-image.

Fortunately, this personal mental solitary confinement usually diminishes with time. But the morale, the psyche, the spirit of the patient becomes extremely depressed. He must be strengthened to be able to offer himself any self-empowerment in healing. Where better to begin this inner journey to rehabilitation than within one's own mind? One day at a time, one step at a time. One breath at a time.

In desperate attempts to survive the ordeal, stroke patients may expend most of their weakened energies without any kind of organized strategy. They are predisposed to become defensive and apologetic to the faceless, judgmental society they live in–and even to their loved ones. Not knowing how to handle this, we waste ourselves, inefficiently trying to regain our perceived diminishment of respect and identity. In this desperate endeavor so much is sacrificed, in pretending not to be different or inadequate. Sadly, stroke patients tend to be all too willing to accept the labels and prejudices foisted on them. And these things often become internalized, and fester within, making the survivor even more flawed–and that adds to his suffering, as well.

We have a profound need to know who we really are, particularly in order to heal from a stroke. The physical can no longer be separated from the spiritual, in this confrontation. But first we must get off the speeding train of blurred perceptions, before we can begin to see ourselves as we truly are. Each of us is an individual with marvelously unique qualities, deserving of self-love and respect. At this grim time, however, it takes a complete change in perspective and attitude for the patient to discern and accept certain personal shocking changes in his reality. After a stroke only the patient can identify and heal what the doctors can't, and what society won't. This ultimate responsibility is the individual's, and no other person can assume it.

Healing entails much more than just medical repairing. It is a very personal and demanding process, as well as an arduous learning experience. It requires the driving responsibility for discovering what is really there, deep inside each of us. Every patient must be self-accountable to create his own particular program, and follow through with it. Yet healing is complex and multifaceted. Our physical realities are only part of our existence. That which is spiritual within us comprises the rest of our being. Thus, recovery requires the healing of one's spirit, as well as one's body.

In the process, stroke survivors must discover their hidden inner resources. During this personal pilgrimage within, it is inevitable that they will experience waves of great triumphs and failures. But during this time they will develop new insights, intimately linked with a sense of intuitive awareness and strength. However long that takes, they eventually will make some contact with the ultimate source of healing that is within each of us. What one does with that can make all the difference. Along with living and growing, healing is a lifelong function. It can only be achieved through a slow and painful personal process of deliberate self-growth and continual commitment to enlightenment–over all prior experience and ego involvement.

The gradual development of self-discovery and self-worth necessitates a unique synthesis of psychological strength and intuitive awareness. The general public's alienation and rejection of the stroke survivor still exists, but that is changing, with increased awareness and education. There eventually comes a time when he must make the choice either to beat the odds, or not. The individual's self-worth must ultimately be defined by himself *as a permanent part of his new social relationship in life*. A whole new psychosocial dimension must be created to eventually enable the stroke survivor to want to take his healing process beyond just the physical restoration of basic functions. This is self-empowerment. This is spirituality.

Case histories show that after a major trauma many patients begin to become more aware of their individual spiritual qualities. One's self is newly perceived as part of a greater whole. Man's will to live is subject to wild extremes, with hope ever ready to germinate, if it is given the opportunity and supportiveness it needs. But the bottom line of defense and healing must come from within oneself. Studies of successful recovery from stroke show a repeated pattern of spiritual growth and self-reliance. This is noticeably missing in the review of patients with only partial recovery.

Historically, Western medicine has treated recovery from stroke or traumatic brain injury on a strictly physical basis. Even today, healing is still looked upon by too many health professionals as limited to considerations concerning somatic damage and repair. That approach has proven shortsighted, and in the final analysis, it is inadequate to total recovery. It views the patient as two-dimensional, without the depth of being and spirituality that are an integral part of one's life.

In recent years, adjuncts to medicine, in the form of individual therapies, have sprung up, as an enlightened need for their services became more apparent. Physical, occupational, speech-language and other therapies have taken great strides in helping satisfy the non-medical needs of patients. Yet these innovations still cannot supplement one of the most basic human requirements of the recovering individual. His sense of self is greatly damaged, and may even be festering. It, too, needs attention and healing. But this is nearly impossible to measure and quantify. Since it can't be reduced to statistics, it is too often discarded by traditional western medicine. In the past, stroke survivors were removed from society. They were comfortably placed well out of sight and mind. Unfortunately, this practice is still with us.

Too often, in traditional treatment the patient is reduced to a medical statistic, and dealt with as such. The first year following a stroke is characterized by attempts to achieve maximum re-training and recovery of former abilities. Yet there are times when the survivor of stroke is made aware that therapy programs can only do so much. Restoration of former physical proficiency most often is left incomplete. These plateaus of maximum physical recovery and development become scary frustrations and barriers to one's healing process. Hope then becomes the most potent medicine for survival and healing, in this frightening valley in the shadow of death. It can open the door to an awareness of our spirituality and strength.

There comes a time when every patient reaches a final plateau in recovery, and is told by the doctors and therapists that his physical dysfunctions will not improve any further. This is so personal and staggering a blow that even many professionals can not comprehend its impact. It is a profound and traumatic experience. All at once, the patient feels abandoned, left without help or hope. The professionals seem to have given up on him, and the psychological impact is overwhelming. At this point the patient is officially pronounced to be a prisoner for life in a dysfunctioning body. This all-too human response is often a depressing outcome of even the best of therapy programs.

When therapy is ended, the recovering patient can hit bottom, emotionally. The depression is terrible, and even suicidal thoughts are not uncommon. He has become a physical misfit in an impatient and confounded society. He feels inferior and defensive, and wants only to remove himself and hide. There is a terrible sense of worthlessness and guilt in imposing himself on others. Despairingly, the patient finally accepts all the negative labels and responses he had fought and rejected, before. Who among us has never experienced moments of the "worthless me" syndrome? But by feeling inferior, the stroke survivor may impede or even reverse the continuation of his own healing process. Intuitively, though, he may begin to realize that there is still much more to healing.

It is a truism that when we sink to the bottom, however terrible it is, the only way to look is up. Case studies show that people recovering from stroke become aware of an inner strength they had never known before. At certain times we have the ability to reach deep within ourselves and come up with an unanticipated perception of hope and personal worth. In a sense, it is like being touched by God. And in this way, stroke survivors can begin to create some order out of the chaos they have to endure.

The healing process must go through torturous but predictable stages. The intense sense of personal loss parallels the psychological reactions one has when grieving the death of a loved one. Indeed, there is bereavement; in a sense, the old self has died. The loss is intense, traumatic and permanent. But this too will pass, if one's potential courage and individual spiritual strength are mustered. All this time the embryo of the new self is growing, waiting and fighting to be born, like the proverbial Phoenix rising from its own ashes.

After generalized stages of anger, denial and depression, overwhelming sense of defeat and victimization, worthless passivity may set in. Patients can feel they will always remain outcasts in society's structure, as well as in their own minds. This is characterized by low self-esteem and a deep, human need for escapist gratification of any kind. Extreme swings in behavior are not uncommon. The recovering patient is very vulnerable at this time. His healing process is on "hold."

This becomes an experience not unlike that of a drug or alcohol addict, who needs sustenance or escape from the subjective realities he finds intolerable. It is interesting to note that all effective recovery programs for addiction also stress a spiritual approach to healing. This step was incorporated into each of these programs because it was found by experience to be the missing element in successful self-rehabilitation. At this point, the stroke survivor may feel too overwhelmed to incorporate the spiritual dimension into his recovery. It may still take some time.

Only well after the initial shock of recognition has passed can the patient learn new things. It takes time and courage to realize that healing requires that one must start all over again, in a *new quest* for personal identity and self-respect. Some survivors are fortunate in coming to this realization by themselves. But most patients need a great deal of external supportiveness and caring direction. Without this they may enter into a period of dejection and hopelessness. They will not try to *make* themselves recover from the psychological trauma inflicted upon them by others, as well as by themselves.

Since a basic part of our humanity is defined by a need for love and nurturing, negative responses can be very disruptive. Depression inhibits healing. The person recovering from a stroke almost always experiences some sense of personal shame and embarrassment. It can be tempting to try to hide one's pain and overwhelming disability, but in the long run, we can't really hide from ourselves.

Chronic illness produces a sense of personal disempowerment. Although it can develop into a psychology of victimization and hopelessness, patients must remember that they have the free will to create something better than what is offered them by others, or by chance. We each have great potentials, within, to offer our self!

For stroke survivors there is still the fate of being cast out of the system. The authorities generalize that whatever healing is possible for them has already been determined by previous data. Thus, the emotionally vulnerable patient can be made into a passive victim by the imposition of a dehumanizing statistical limitation. But hope is always the great healer, and it can be revived to counter many afflictions. Without hope, healing is diminished or even proscribed.

We have learned that recovery requires overcoming apathy and depression. It involves learning to integrate and live with one's physical disability. The only alternative would be to suffer permanently, which would prevent any further inner development. But even during the worst of times, our natural senses generate gut-level signals. We grow by learning to understand the dimensions of our dreams, doubts, fears and frustrations–and work through them. Although the individual is physically limited, his spirit still can soar. The ultimate decision and empowerment come from within. One's body may be encumbered, but his humanity and animating principle may be even more functional than before. Unfortunately, some stay with the negative option, and remain mired in self-pity and isolation, or even rage, for the rest of their lives. Yet everyone has that remarkable choice: to heal themselves, or not.

Amazingly, just as a negative self-image retards healing, a positive one abets it. But to maximize recovery, one must be concerned with much more than just the physical aspects of rehabilitation. The energy, quality of life and spirit of the individual need to be self-acknowledged and endorsed. This requires finding new or different pathways, including ones that were presumed to be closed. Ultimately, healing is very much influenced by hope and spiritual development.

Recovery, beyond physical healing, demands abandoning old patterns or strategies. It is about discovery of new directions of creativity, and new doors that the individual can open on life. It requires a great desire to be whole, and a refusal to be a victim of circumstance and statistics. This springs from hope and self-reliance, but recovery means going through a painful learning process, and being wrung through the full gamut of intense emotions. As with any other major psychological traumas, it is necessary to confront and experience the fears, anxieties, limitations and even humiliations that lie in wait, in order to get past them.

Healing is abetted by attending to the instructions of intuition. These can be misunderstood, but they are never false. They may be masked by anxieties and fears, at first, and one may mistake these emotions for the underlying instinct. Intuition, however, does not involve judgment, memory, fact or intellect. It is the inborn wisdom of our collective unconscious speaking to each of us, asking to be recognized.

Intuition is a fundamental and instinctive function of the human being. It is as basic as the native wisdom of birds in migration. How do they understand what to do, except for their inborn intuition or instinct? Undoubtedly, they don't really comprehend their actions, as we define comprehension. Animals naturally feel and follow their unchallenged inner instincts. Thus, they are at one with nature, and without the artificial constructs that we create for our own species. Too often our daily struggles for achievement, recognition and material gain can blind us to the beauty and wisdom of the intuition inherent within us.

Ironically, disability can be the means to step away from the masks and other artificial impediments that restrict us. We are forced to create and adapt new methods that will work for us in this dark, uncharted territory. Instinct can offer us the insight to strip off the deceptive and stressful outer layers of living. It can reveal the pure self. Indeed, healing is stimulated when one realizes that after a stroke he still has his basic self, complete with instinct, intuition and hope.

Yet it is so hard to be independent of the influences of a caring yet ignorant and sometimes insensitive society. What is of prime importance to the stroke recoverer is his immediate situation and eventual recovery. It is so difficult at times to be patient and take things on a day-by-day basis. One can easily lose perspective of the great strides he has already taken, in the agonizingly slow process of healing. But when we have been forced through the worst, we can become more sensitized to the intangible, subconscious perception available to each of us. By embracing our intuitive strength and wisdom we can learn to handle more effectively whatever comes our way. In realizing the need for this self-reliance, we lay the foundation for self-empowerment in healing.

Not surprisingly, a sense of humor is a powerful healing medicine. It is also a necessary component of a healthy and balanced way of life. When we can laugh without bitterness at ourselves, and others, it is a sure sign of healing. Although the physical damage can not be repaired beyond a given point, in the final analysis, psychic damage can be completely self-healed if the passion is strong enough. Even extreme disability can not deprive us of our inner heritage. It is very ironic, but surviving a stroke can become the cardinal turning-point in one's ever-evolving awareness and growth.

It is impossible to speculate as to how many perfect physical human bodies house incomplete or unhappy spirits. Engulfed in superficiality, many people take too much for granted, and well may have lost their sense of wonder. They have not known a new pathway in a very long time, and are no longer enthusiastic or excited. They have lost elan. Very little seems inspiring or interesting. Even individuals with healthy bodies do not realize that what they need most is often hidden from them. Yet all the while it is inside, ever within their grasp. In sharp contrast, there are so many people with physical disabilities who are excited and appreciative of everything in their lives. That is the essence of recovery! But it requires an understanding and love of more than just the physical self.

We are reared with social attitudes that label adversity and pain as negative concepts. But the individual who recovers from severe illness eventually learns that these conditions are not necessarily bad. In the recovery process one must go through many experiences, but one must first identify and accept one's inner self and no longer embrace the role of victim. Identifying the real source of emotional distress is essential to its elimination. Genuine recovery starts when we stop wallowing in self-pity. At this point we make room for good thoughts to enter our lives. In contrast to permanent physical debilitation, we can continually heal and grow beyond any degree of psychic disability. Our humanity can continue to grow within us, as long as we are able to draw breath. We discover that this can be an amazing life, full of wonders and possibilities.

Despite any physical disability, each of us is whole in the center of his being. Nobody is without some kind of impairment, emotional or physical. But within the marvel of our minds, every one of us has the innate ability to self-heal. This must be appreciated by our intellects, as well as our hearts. We may be stuck with the physical package that is dealt us, but our minds are not limited. Missing a limb or even a string of physical functions is not nearly as incapacitating as being without heart and spirit. That is real disability. Ultimately, each of us is a projection of his own spirit, and we can go on striving for what we want to become. Stroke and physical impediment can not prevent this growth.

When we are isolated from our former lives by extreme illness and infirmity we have a chance to see things in new ways. But whether or not we do depends completely on our individual makeup. Hope and a sense of personal spirituality keep us going, despite depression, desperation and pessimism that sometimes interfere and prey so heavily on us.

Hope is a natural outer expression of our innate inner self. When there seems to be nothing left, all that we have remaining is this precious shard of life. To live, we must have hope. The everyday tasks and plans for tomorrow are not enough. We must move on, refusing to dwell on the labels and plateaus of our physical limitations. The essential quality of hope brings us into closer touch with our inner humanity and spirit. It is a means to discover our true potentials.

Although some truths may be very painful to accept, they offer us lessons. Confusion and chaos can seem to be running things, especially while one is going through the extraordinary and largely subjective processes of recovery from stroke. It is normal to feel sadness or even depression at never being able to regain a life that is lost. Everywhere, one encounters doubts, conflicting opinions and suggestions, and in despair, one ponders what to believe. But the ultimate perception must come from a deep place within one's self–it is the fountainhead of real healing.

We are all on this mysterious journey, together, yet, paradoxically, we are each alone. This is wonderful and ever-evolving. But in the final analysis, nobody can tell anyone else its meaning. Unavoidably, each of us must learn, to whatever degree he or she is willing or capable, the extent of life's intimate values. The answers as well as the right questions are here, but they are hidden in personal metaphors of cosmic proportion. The questions first must be identified to be of any value. The answers are as elemental and simple as they are universal and profound. We can find them by departing from the all-too-familiar conventional methods that have proved to be inadequate. This deeply existential quest is the most intensely personal pilgrimage one can make. But the rewards are enriching, beyond anything else in life.

When delving into this inner space we are completely alone with ourselves. At first, that can be frightening; we are forced to come face-to-face with the fragment of godhead that is part of each of us. We are thrown entirely upon our own inner resources. From this the realization grows that we can not honestly blame others or outside events for our own failures or setbacks. What we are and what we will become depends so much on what is learned from our inner selves. In our inner human growth nothing is truly impossible. Healing is only part of this potential within us.

There are so many examples of disabled people who *made* life happen for them. This includes Demosthenes, Helen Keller and a very impressive list of celebrities, too long to be listed here. And there also must have been so very many others, too unobtrusive to be examples for inspiration. What did they learn that we have yet to find out? Certainly, it was not something that they only subjectively imagined. Whatever it was, it had to be real enough to work for them! Surely, there is an important lesson to be learned from this.

Disability has enough of its own limitations, but it should never be allowed to define the person within. Among the most remarkable illustrations of this idea is the case of Stephen Hawking, a paraplegic, suffering from severe ALS, who many say is even more brilliant than Einstein. Had he allowed his terrible multiple physical afflictions to limit or define him, modern physics would be much the poorer, today. The world of scientific knowledge is advanced regularly with his extraordinary contributions.

Despite his twisted dysfunctional body, his beautiful life should be an inspiration to everyone, particularly those who also have serious disabilities. He did not dissolve in self-pity, but remained his own person, in defiance of the nearly impossible handicaps that would have crushed most others. His extensive physical disability, almost unbelievable in its severity and scope, could not stop his mind from working. And despite the unimaginable, nearly total deterioration of his body, that mind is undoubtedly getting even better than it was before. He *makes* it continue to grow and serve him and the rest of civilization. He is our valiant brother and teacher.

We are inspired by his example. He shows us that just *coping* with severe illness and disability is not nearly enough. We must go beyond that which afflicts us, and create ways to heal ourselves, and grow, again. We can learn to celebrate the human spirit within each of us.

Since time immemorial we have been conditioned to view suffering as a thoroughly bad thing. Thus, we are conditionally blinded to any of the benefits that, somehow, might be attained from it. In self-empowerment, we learn to stop denying the negative stresses that restrict us, and actually embrace them—enabling ourselves to *work through* them. Indeed, "Sweet are the uses of adversity." With a single-minded commitment to a higher purpose, we become capable of transforming even the horror of disability into a positive means for self-growth. The survivor recovering from the havoc of stroke can become a far better person *because of* this unwanted suffering and ironic twist of fate.

Each of us has a great potential for healing and achievement. The body/mind response that powers the "placebo effect" has been vastly underrated and misunderstood. Possibly, it should be called something else, to remove any possible negative associations—perhaps something positive, like "self-empowerment healing" or "mind/body healing." Regardless of what it is called, it is a marvelous expression of our humanity, and should not be denied. We can and should apply this remarkable healing principle in each of our lives, regardless of any degree of physical disability.

As mentioned earlier, the word "spirituality" often is incorrectly comprehended. Some people too hastily assign it meanings linked to the occult or to aspects of overzealous religion. But nothing could be farther from the truth. Spiritual values are our most precious possessions. They deal directly with our most personal perceptions of existence, ultimate meaning, and even God. What could be more profound?

Discovering spiritual awareness and expression enables each individual to evolve to a higher step, despite lifelong, built-up layers of distraction and confusion. In this paradox we begin to comprehend why we are worth far more than that which our physical disabilities would dictate. Each of us can be empowered, through a spiritual approach to healing, to live *with* physical disability, and grow–rather than suffer and stagnate *from* it, as before. In this way we can take the power away from disability and give it to ourselves.

In self-healing we emerge from the barriers and blocks that can diminish our individualism and achievement. We learn more fully to integrate life, rather than continue to stagnate in a private, painful, fragmented existence. Self-healing provides us with the inner strength to grow out of the cocoon-like life space we all too often tend to weave for ourselves. This enables us to reject the limiting concept of coping with adversity–*and go beyond it.*

Each of us has the amazing potential to become self-empowered–to recognize and change the external as well as the internal myths that keep us imprisoned. It is a strange irony, but after the stroke experience, many wonderful things about life may be discovered, that otherwise may not have been. We discover how to heal, one step at a time, while establishing positive control over conditions that could have become a permanent tragedy. In effect, through the discovery and appreciation of the spiritual self, we change and enrich our total life experience.

In taking charge and responsibility for his own healing and developing, the stroke recoverer can actually create his own metamorphosis. Like the phoenix rising from its own ashes, a *new* person is waiting to be born. With the development of self-empowerment it becomes possible to grow again, better and better, and to celebrate the marvels of the healing human spirit within each of us.

Index

Note: Page numbers preceded by *mentioned* indicates intermittent discussion of the subject on each inclusive page.

265

Pain
  and suffering, distinctions of,
    130,131,133
  stroke-related
    and muscular spasticity, 76
    pre-onset headaches and, 9,
      10,17,151-152
    psychiatric implications for, 17
Palm Springs Stroke Activity Center,
    227-231
Paralysis; hemiplegia, 47. *See also*
    Motor ability/mobility;
    Muscular weakness;
    Physical therapy
  occupational therapy for, 115-117
  as rehab patient selection
    criterion, 29-31
  stroke effects toward causing, 8
  and thalamic pain syndrome, 17
Paranoia, 19
Parietal lobe syndrome, 17
Pat and Roald (Farrell), 191. *See also*
    Neal, Patricia
Pathophysiology of stroke, 7-13
  definitions of stroke, 15,21
  of clinical classifications of,
    7-8. *See also specific*
    classifications and types of
    strokes
  frequency, 10-11
  impairments and acute
    disabilities, 8-9,24,
    46-47,99. *See also specific*
    impairments and relevant
    therapies
  incidence. *See* Incidence of stroke
    and stroke-related factors
  mortality rates, 9,10,11,252
    and survival rates, 222,225,231
  and pathology emphasized in
    treatment and rehab,
    46,254,256,259
  prevalence, 10,11
  risk factors, 11-13,16. *See also*
    specific risks

sites of lesions/infarcts. *See* Brain
    areas
  symptoms. *See* Symptoms and
    warning signs
Personality factors, as stroke risk, 16
Perceptual impairments. *See* Visual
    impairments; *specific*
    impairments; see under
    Psychological studies
Pet therapy, 175-176,229
Physiatrists, 50,51,94,228
Physical therapy; therapists, 50,
    51-52,201,201,228,229,
    241,242
  compensatory techniques and
    devices, 24,112,116-117,122
  discharge planning, 113
  evaluation of patient, 109-111
  and family participation and
    training in, 110-111,112-113
  goal setting and program
    planning, 110-111
  interdisciplinary communication,
    110,111
  techniques for reversal/prevention
    of stroke effects, 111-112
Physicians. *See also specific*
    specialties
  emphasis on physical stroke
    recovery by medical science
    and, 46,254,256,259
  suffering caused by medical
    science and, 132,134,141
  and inadequately viewed by,
    130-131,134,139,141
Post-Stroke Consultation Service,
    48-56
Post-traumatic stress disorder
    (PTSD), 155-156
Prevalence of stroke, 10,11. *See also*
    Incidence of stroke
Procedure Manual in Speech
    Pathology with
    Brain-Damaged Adults, A
    (Keenan), 191

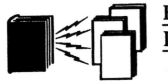

Haworth
DOCUMENT DELIVERY
SERVICE

This valuable service provides a single-article order form for any article from a Haworth journal.

- *Time Saving:* No running around from library to library to find a specific article.
- *Cost Effective:* All costs are kept down to a minimum.
- *Fast Delivery:* Choose from several options, including same-day FAX.
- *No Copyright Hassles:* You will be supplied by the original publisher.
- *Easy Payment:* Choose from several easy payment methods.

Open Accounts Welcome for . . .
- Library Interlibrary Loan Departments
- Library Network/Consortia Wishing to Provide Single-Article Services
- Indexing/Abstracting Services with Single Article Provision Services
- Document Provision Brokers and Freelance Information Service Providers

MAIL or *FAX* THIS ENTIRE ORDER FORM TO:

Haworth Document Delivery Service
The Haworth Press, Inc.
10 Alice Street
Binghamton, NY 13904-1580

or FAX: 1-800-895-0582
or CALL: 1-800-342-9678
9am-5pm EST

PLEASE SEND ME PHOTOCOPIES OF THE FOLLOWING SINGLE ARTICLES:

1) Journal Title: _____
   Vol/Issue/Year: _____ Starting & Ending Pages: _____
   Article Title: _____
   _____

2) Journal Title: _____
   Vol/Issue/Year: _____ Starting & Ending Pages: _____
   Article Title: _____
   _____

3) Journal Title: _____
   Vol/Issue/Year: _____ Starting & Ending Pages: _____
   Article Title: _____
   _____

4) Journal Title: _____
   Vol/Issue/Year: _____ Starting & Ending Pages: _____
   Article Title: _____

(See other side for Costs and Payment Information)

COSTS: Please figure your cost to order quality copies of an article.

1. Set-up charge per article: $8.00
   ($8.00 × number of separate articles)   _____

2. Photocopying charge for each article:
   1-10 pages: $1.00   _____

   11-19 pages: $3.00   _____

   20-29 pages: $5.00   _____

   30+ pages: $2.00/10 pages   _____

3. Flexicover (optional): $2.00/article   _____

4. Postage & Handling: US: $1.00 for the first article/
   $.50 each additional article   _____

   Federal Express: $25.00   _____

   Outside US: $2.00 for first article/
   $.50 each additional article _____

5. Same-day FAX service: $.35 per page   _____

GRAND TOTAL: _____

METHOD OF PAYMENT: (please check one)

❑ Check enclosed   ❑ Please ship and bill. PO # _____
   (sorry we can ship and bill to bookstores only! All others must pre-pay)

❑ Charge to my credit card: ❑ Visa; ❑ MasterCard; ❑ Discover;
   ❑ American Express;

Account Number: _____ Expiration date:_____

Signature: ✗_____

Name: _____ Institution: _____

Address: _____

_____

City: _____ State:_____ Zip:_____

Phone Number: _____ FAX Number: _____

MAIL or *FAX* THIS ENTIRE ORDER FORM TO:

Haworth Document Delivery Service	**or FAX:** 1-800-895-0582
The Haworth Press, Inc.	**or CALL:** 1-800-342-9678
10 Alice Street	9am-5pm EST)
Binghamton, NY 13904-1580	